Cardiology
 **IN** *focus*

Glyn Thomas MRCP

British Heart Foundation Research Fellow
Department of Biochemistry
University of Cambridge
Specialist Registrar in Cardiology
St Bartholomew's Hospital, London

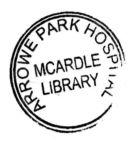

Peter M Schofield MD FRCP FACC

Consultant Cardiologist
Papworth Hospital, Cambridge

Andrew A Grace PhD FRCP FACC

Consultant Cardiologist
Papworth Hospital, Cambridge
Senior Research Fellow, University of Cambridge

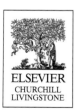

ELSEVIER
CHURCHILL
LIVINGSTONE

EDINBURGH   LONDON   NEW YORK   OXFORD   PHILADELPHIA   ST LOUIS   SYDNEY   TORONTO 2005

ELSEVIER | CHURCHILL
LIVINGSTONE
An imprint of Elsevier Limited

First published as Colour Guide Cardiology 1993
Second edition 1997
    Reprinted 1998
First In Focus edition 2005

ISBN 0443074232

British Library Cataloguing in Publication Data
A catalogue record for this book is available from the British Library

Library of Congress Cataloging in Publication Data
A catalog record for this book is available from the Library of Congress

Note
Medical knowledge is constantly changing. Standard safety precautions must be followed, but
as new research and clinical experience broaden our knowledge, changes in treatment and
drug therapy may become necessary or appropriate. Readers are advised to check the most
current product information provided by the manufacturer of each drug to be administered
to verify the recommended dose, the method and duration of administration, and
contraindications. It is the responsibility of the practitioner, relying on experience and
knowledge of the patient, to determine dosages and the best treatment for each individual
patient. Neither the publisher nor the authors assumes any liability for any injury and/or
damage to persons or property arising from this publication.

 **your source for books,
journals and multimedia
in the health sciences**
www.elsevierhealth.com

The
publisher's
policy is to use
**paper manufactured
from sustainable forests**

Printed in China

Cardiology

For Elsevier

Commissioning Editor: Laurence Hunter
Project Development Manager: Helen Leng
Project Manager: Frances Affleck
Design Direction: George Ajayi

Preface

The purpose of the book is to give a broad and balanced overview of modern practice for those who manage patients with cardiovascular disease. The complex interplay occurring between the bedside, and high technology should be seen as a key theme.

In the task of collecting images for the book we have received invaluable help, as previously, from numerous colleagues. These individuals in particular deserve our special thanks: Dr Jim Hall and Dr Martin Lowe, co-authors for previous related works, have been, as usual, generous in their support and Dr Hugh Fleming, Senior Consultant Cardiologist, Papworth Hospital, 1959–1988, deserves our thanks for the photographs of his patients that were used extensively in his clinical teaching. Our colleagues and friends from Papworth Hospital, Cambridge, and elsewhere have generously provided illustrations and include: Professor Bob Anderson, Mr Stephen Large, Dr Michael Petch, Dr Len Shapiro, Dr David Stone, Dr Edward Rowland, Dr Hugh Bethell, Dr K Ranjadayalan, Dr Abdul Suliman, Dr Fred Foo, Dr Neha Sekhri, Dr A Deauer and Mrs. E Gorman. Finally, special thanks to Dr L Cunningham.

Contents

Many factors have been identified that influence the progression of coronary atherosclerosis.

Major risk factors include male sex, increasing age, smoking, hyperlipidaemia, hypertension and diabetes mellitus. Minor risk factors include family history of coronary artery disease, sedentary lifestyle/obesity, excessive alcohol consumption, haemostatic factors (elevated fibrinogen, factor VII, plasminogen activator inhibitor 1, homocysteine levels), biochemical markers, elevated CRP and psychological stress (type A personality).

Smoking

The risk of myocardial infarction in smokers is three times that of non-smokers. The use of cigarettes leads to an unfavourable alteration in high-density lipoprotein (HDL) cholesterol structure and function as well as a direct effect on coronary vasomotor tone. Smoking multiplies the negative effect of other risk factors.

Hyper-lipidaemia

Raised plasma lipids are due to a combination of genetic and environmental factors. Elevated low-density lipoprotein (LDL) has been implicated as the most significant dyslipidaemia implicated in coronary heart disease. In familial hypercholesterolaemia the gene that encodes the LDL receptor is either reduced in number or dysfunctional, leading to reduced clearance of LDL cholesterol from the plasma. Heterozygotes (incidence approximately 1:500) have elevated plasma cholesterol often up to 15 mmol/l. Homozygotes (incidence approximately 1:1 000 000) may have massively increased plasma cholesterol values, e.g. 15–30 mmol/l. Clinical features include corneal arcus, xanthelasma and tendon xanthomata. The benefits of statin therapy are now well established in heterozygotes.

Hypertension

Hypertension is established as a strong independent risk factor for coronary heart disease, leading to a twofold increase in risk. Drug treatment of isolated mild to moderate hypertension can reduce the risk of both myocardial infarction (15%) and stroke (40%). The greatest cardiovascular benefit of blood pressure control is seen in those patients with other risk factors, e.g. diabetes mellitus.

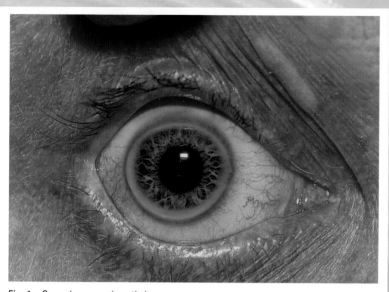

Fig. 1 Corneal arcus and xanthelasma.

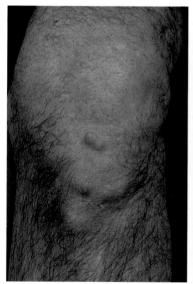

Fig. 2 Lipid deposition around the patella in type III hypercholesterolaemia.

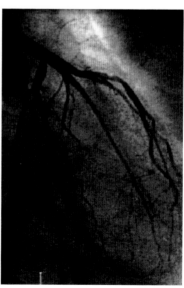

Fig. 3 Left coronary arteriogram from young patient with homozygousFH showing diffuse coronary disease.

Angina pectoris is the symptomatic manifestation of myocardial ischaemia. Angina is most frequently described as a central substernal dull ache with radiation to the jaw and left arm. The most important feature to establish in the history is the relationship to exercise. The rapid resolution of symptoms on stopping exertion or with sublingual nitroglycerin is often the most important clue obtained from the clinical history. However the diagnosis should never be considered simple: atypical chest pain is common and often difficult to distinguish from true angina.

Terminology

Chronic stable angina pectoris
Typical symptoms are predictably brought on by exercise or stress, particularly in cold weather or after a heavy meal. Symptoms occur when myocardial oxygen demand outstrips supply, usually because of a fixed atheromatous narrowing impairing flow in one or more of the coronary arteries.

Acute coronary syndrome
This term encompasses the clinical consequence of an 'unstable' plaque within the coronary artery. Plaque rupture may not necessarily lead to ST segment elevation and Q wave formation; hence this situation, formerly called unstable angina pectoris, is termed non-ST elevation acute coronary syndrome (NSTEACS). Angina occurs in a rapidly progressive pattern at rest or on minimal exertion. A proportion of these patients will develop a subsequent elevation in biochemical markers of cellular damage, termed non-ST elevation myocardial infarction (NSTEMI). NSTEACS may occur as a result of changes in tone within the coronary arteries. This uncommon condition is referred to as variant or Prinzmetal's angina. Symptoms are identical to those of NSTEACS.

Pathology

Coronary narrowing due to atheroma is the most common cause of angina pectoris, with symptoms usually appearing when coronary artery lesions become 'critical' (>70% stenosis). Pathological studies, however, emphasize that even in the presence of most such lesions patients may be asymptomatic, the initial manifestation being sudden death.

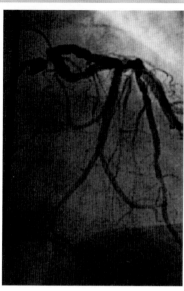

Fig. 4 Coronary arteriogram showing severe left main stem stenosis.

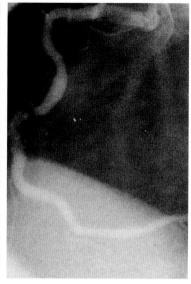

Fig. 5 Coronary stenosis in mid right coronary artery.

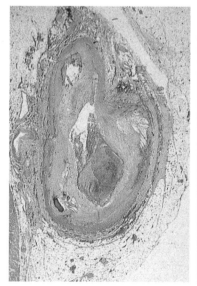

Fig. 6 Histological cross-section of an atheromatous plaque with luminal thrombus.

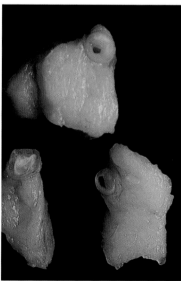

Fig. 7 Transverse sections through the three coronary arteries showing severe three-vessel disease.

3 Coronary heart disease syndromes: angina pectoris

Initial investigations

Electrocardiography

The initial assessment of the patient with symptoms suggestive of angina pectoris should include an ECG. In most patients with uncomplicated angina the ECG is normal or there are minor repolarization changes such as ST segment depression or T wave inversion. Pathological Q waves may be present, indicating prior transmural myocardial infarction. Features of left ventricular hypertrophy may suggest associated hypertension or aortic stenosis.

Chest X–ray

This investigation is of low value in the patient with coronary heart disease, although other important conditions may be revealed, such as calcification of the aortic valve (best seen on a lateral film) seen in aortic valve stenosis.

Echocardiography

Extremely valuable in the assessment of left ventricular function, and to investigate the possibility of valvular disease.

Biochemistry/haematology

Markers of myocardial cell injury such as creatinine kinase and troponin I/T are not raised in stable angina pectoris. Elevation in these markers would usually require inpatient investigation and treatment as an acute coronary syndrome. A fasting cholesterol profile should be obtained and lipid-lowering therapy commenced if the cholesterol is raised. A full blood count to exclude anaemia and thyroid function tests should be considered.

Further assessment

In most patients further investigations are required to establish the presence of underlying coronary artery disease and to stratify risk. These may be non-invasive, usually involving some form of stress testing to establish the presence of reversible myocardial ischaemia. Invasive testing with coronary angiography can indicate both the presence and the extent of coronary artery disease. New techniques under evaluation include electron beam computed tomography (EBCT) and magnetic resonance imaging (MRI).

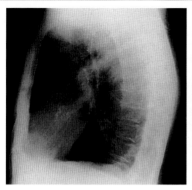

Fig. 8 Lateral chest X-ray in aortic stenosis showing valvar calcification.

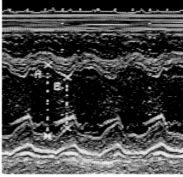

Fig. 9 M-mode echocardiogram, left ventricle showing impaired contraction.

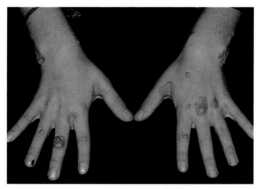

Fig. 10 Extensive planar xanthomata in familial hypercholesterolaemia.

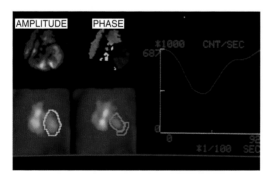

Fig. 11 Gated nuclear ventriculogram (MUGA) showing normal function (ejection fraction (EF) 53%) in a patient with angina.

Exercise electrocardiography

Indications

1. Further investigation of patients with moderate risk of coronary artery disease and normal resting ECG. Sensitivity only ≈70%, so a negative test does not exclude the diagnosis. 2. Can provide information on functional capacity and prognosis in patients with known angina. 3. Risk stratification following MI. 4. Provocation of arrhythmia in patients with palpitations provoked by exertion. 5. Risk stratification in patients with hypertrophic cardiomyopathy.

Contra-indications

Most ambulant patients are capable of sufficient exercise (>85% age-predicted maximum heart rate) to obtain a clinically useful result. Patients with unstable coronary disease, uncontrolled hypertension, severe aortic stenosis or pulmonary hypertension are usually considered unsuitable.

Method

Exercise level is gradually increased on a motorized treadmill or bicycle ergometer. Specific protocols are described to allow comparison between centres and over time, e.g. the Bruce protocol. Concomitant antianginal therapy, especially beta-blockers, are known to reduce the sensitivity of the test; therefore sometimes omitted for 2–3 days before, dependent on context.

Interpretation

In addition to the ECG, symptoms and blood pressure response to exercise are observed. The test is terminated on reaching the predetermined end-point (maximum heart rate), symptoms of chest pain, ST changes or the provocation of arrhythmia. The principal ECG change indicating a positive response is planar or down-sloping depression of the ST segment >0.1 mV (1 mm). In the presence of typical anginal chest discomfort, the predictive value for coronary artery disease is greater than 90%.

Myocardial perfusion imaging

Myocardial perfusion imaging employs exercise or pharmacological stress, e.g. with intravenous adenosine or dobutamine to provoke ischaemia. The isotope is injected at peak stress and its myocardial distribution relates to coronary flow. These tests can distinguish ischaemic (reversible defect) and infarcted tissue (irreversible defect) from normal tissue by the pattern of isotope distribution detected by a gamma camera. Such investigations are indicated when there is diagnostic doubt following an exercise ECG, in patients with an abnormal resting ECG in whom changes on exercise are not interpretable (e.g. bundle branch block, LVH) and in patients who are unable to exercise (e.g. peripheral vascular disease, osteoarthritis).

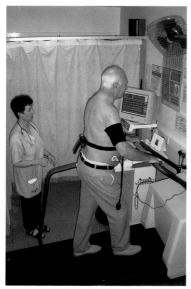

Fig. 12 Patient with leads attached ready for treadmill exercise test.

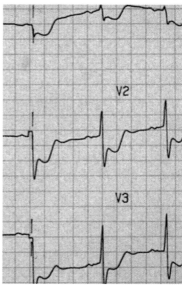

Fig. 13 Planar ST depression indicating myocardial ischaemia.

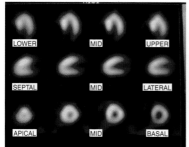

Fig. 14 Exercise perfusion study (rest image) showing normal perfusion.

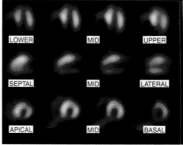

Fig. 15 Exercise perfusion study (exercise image) showing impaired segmental inferior perfusion.

Coronary arteriography

With the development of effective non-invasive methods of assessing the presence and extent of ischaemia cardiac catheterization is now principally indicated in patients with presumptive coronary artery disease to assess the extent of disease and to define a strategy for revascularization. The development of percutaneous transluminal coronary angioplasty has widened the requirement for the technique and well in excess of 1 million procedures are performed annually in the USA.

Indications

Establishing the diagnosis   In patients with atypical symptoms of angina pectoris and equivocal non-invasive investigations, arteriography provides the only established method of defining the diagnosis.

Determining prognosis   In patients with easily provoked angina including those with post-MI pain, the prognosis is principally determined by the extent of coronary disease and left ventricular function and will be defined by angiography.

Planning therapy   In patients who have an inadequate response to drug therapy, arteriography determines the most appropriate approach to revascularization.

Technique

The procedure is carried out under local anaesthetic. Arterial access is usually obtained via femoral or radial artery puncture or by cutdown onto the brachial artery. Preshaped catheters are used to selectively intubate the origins of the coronary arteries and enter the left ventricular cavity. Contrast solution is injected through the lumen of the catheter and digital or cine images are obtained. The procedure usually takes around 10–15 minutes and is well tolerated by the majority of patients.

Complications

The incidence of major complications is now low, with a mortality of about 0.06%. Most of the relatively minor complications are produced at the site of vascular access (local complications).

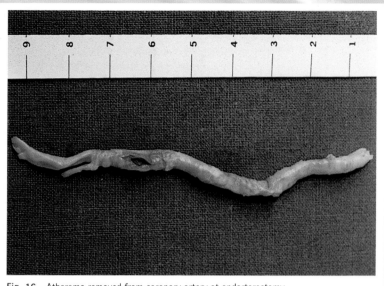

Fig. 16 Atheroma removed from coronary artery at endarterectomy.

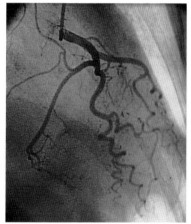

Fig. 17 Left coronary arteriogram.

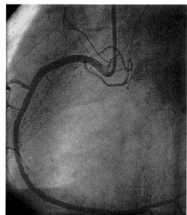

Fig. 18 Right coronary arteriogram.

Medical treatment

The main objectives are symptom relief, prognostic improvement and risk factor control. All patients require lifestyle advice, which includes smoking cessation, healthy eating (may include weight loss and a reduction in salt intake if indicated) and regular aerobic exercise. Hyperlipidaemia should be treated by dietary measures, and lipid-lowering agents are usually required. Aspirin reduces the risk of myocardial infarction and should be given to all patients in the absence of contraindications. Beta-blockers reduce heart rate and oxygen demand, thus alleviating symptoms of angina. They also reduce the incidence of myocardial infarction and sudden death in selected patients. Further medical therapy includes sublingual and long-acting oral nitrates and calcium channel blockers. Patients whose symptoms continue or who have prognostically severe disease are candidates for revascularization with either percutaneous coronary intervention or bypass surgery.

Percutaneous intervention (PCI)

Procedure

These procedures like cardiac catheterization, are performed under local anaesthetic. A fine guide wire is passed through the coronary catheter and down the coronary artery across the narrowing. A balloon catheter is passed over the guide wire and inflated, compressing the atheroma and dilating the artery, thus relieving the obstruction. A stent is usually placed.

Results

Successful reduction of a coronary stenosis usually relieves angina. Studies comparing PCI with coronary bypass surgery indicate no real prognostic difference but a greater need for further revascularization procedures with PCI.

Complications

The mortality following PCI is now low (<<1%) but acute reocclusion of the dilated artery remains a serious problem. In 20–30% of patients, restenosis of the dilated vessel occurred 1–6 months following PCI prior to the use of stents/drug elution.

Coronary Stenting

Coronary stents are metallic coils or slotted tubular structures delivered at the site of the coronary artery stenosis by balloon inflation. Used in conjunction with balloon angioplasty, stents reduce angina recurrence, restenosis (by ≈15–20%) and consequently the need for further PCI and coronary surgery. Although particularly useful in acute occlusion, coronary dissection, restenosis and vein graft

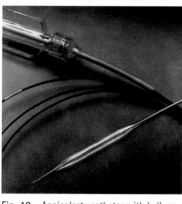

Fig. 19 Angioplasty catheter with balloon inflated.

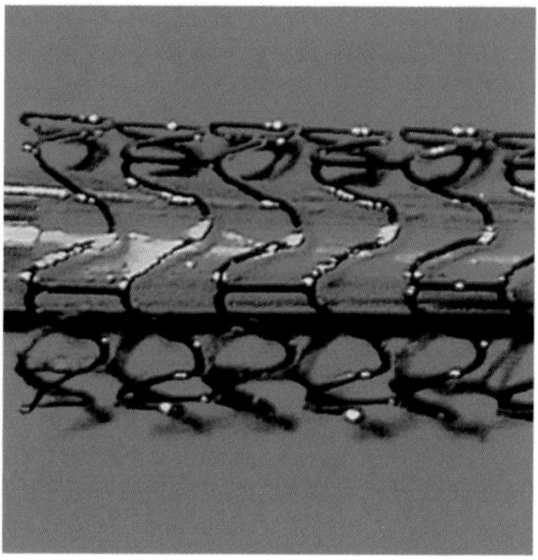

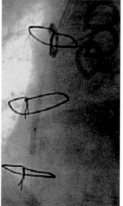

Fig. 20 Coronary stent.

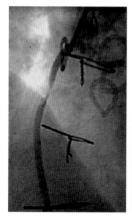

Fig. 21 Right coronary vein graft with severe stenosis.

Fig. 22 Angioplasty balloon inflated at site of stenosis.

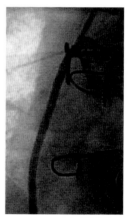

Fig. 23 Following balloon inflation the graft is widely patent.

disease, their use is almost universal. Drug-eluting stents are now available, allowing even greater patency rates. The main risk of stent deployment is thrombotic occlusion, seen in around 4% of patients within 2 weeks.

Coronary artery bypass surgery (CABG)

Indications

Relief of symptoms   CABG is an effective method of relieving angina with >90% success rate. In the USA patients with relatively mild symptoms have historically received such surgery whereas in Europe typical surgical cases have had disabling symptoms or have been intolerant of medical therapy. CABG is one of the most common operative procedures undertaken in the USA.

Improvement of prognosis   Patients with left main stem disease and some with triple vessel disease have an improved prognosis following CABG. Contraindications to surgery are diminishing but risk increases with impaired left ventricular function and coexistent medical problems, especially cerebrovascular disease.

Procedure

The left internal mammary artery (LIMA) is now the graft conduit of choice. Usually it is used for grafting one vessel, e.g. the left anterior descending (LAD) artery. The vessel is dissected free of the sternum and connected to the coronary artery distal to the stenosis. Most patients require multiple bypasses and lengths of the saphenous vein have traditionally been used. The grafts are anastomosed to the aortic root and then to the distal segment of the diseased coronary arteries. Radial arteries are also used and have superior patency rates to veins.

Risks

Perioperative mortality ($\approx$1–2%) is not declining, as patients with more preoperative risk factors become surgical candidates. Morbidity is low with the risk of significant postbypass cerebral impairment being small.

Follow-up

Coronary surgery remains palliative in the treatment of coronary disease. Patients require careful follow-up with particular attention to secondary prevention, especially smoking cessation and lipid management. All should receive life-long aspirin. Saphenous vein graft occlusion is inevitable and only lessened by these manoeuvres. Arterial grafts show a strikingly higher patency rate with prolonged relief of angina and improved prognosis.

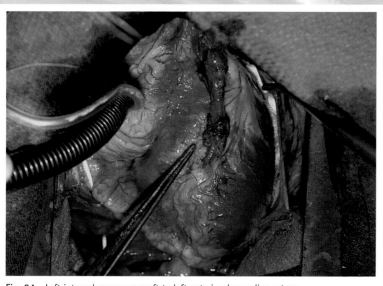

Fig. 24 Left internal mammary graft to left anterior descending artery.

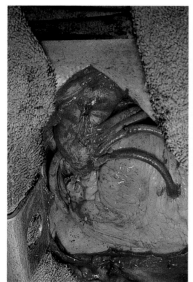

Fig. 26 Angiogram showing stenosed coronary artery saphenous vein graft.

Fig. 25 Multiple saphenous vein grafts in situ.

4 Non-ST-elevation acute coronary syndrome (NSTEACS)

Definition

Clinical syndrome that incorporates the groups of patients previously classified as having unstable angina, or non-Q wave (subendocardial) myocardial infarction. Presentation consists of angina that is new, occurs at rest or is rapidly progressive.

Pathology

The underlying pathology is ulceration or rupture of an atheromatous plaque. Microembolization of platelet aggregates can lead to myocardial damage of varying severity. Cytokines are released, increasing smooth muscle tone with vasoconstriction further reducing flow.

Investigations

Electrocardiography An ECG during an episode of pain will often show ST depression with or without T wave inversion. Occasionally other patterns develop, such as T wave peaking or bundle branch block.

Biochemical markers Microemboli may lead to a disruption of the myocyte membrane and release of intracellular contents. A rise in creatinine kinase (CK–MB) greater than three times the upper limit of normal is diagnostic of myocardial infarction. These emboli may, however, lead to a microinfarct, where no CK–MB rise is detected. In this situation, measurement of relatively cardiac-specific troponins (TnT or TnI) may reveal evidence of myocardial necrosis. An estimated 30% of patients with pain and ECG changes without a CK–MB rise are diagnosed as non-ST-elevation myocardial infarction (NSTEMI) by troponin assay.

Management

Antiplatelet therapy consists of aspirin and clopidogrel. Anticoagulation is most conveniently provided by subcutaneous low-molecular-weight (LMW) heparin. Symptom control is gained by the use of beta-blockers, calcium antagonists and oral/intravenous nitrates with continued pain, especially with ECG changes and/or positive troponins, intravenous GP IIb/IIIa receptor antagonists (e.g. tirofiban, abciximab) can be used. These drugs are of particular benefit to those patients who then undergo PCI. There is no role for thrombolysis in NSTEACS. Following resolution of symptoms, those patients with positive troponins, or negative troponins with positive exercise test, will require coronary angiography.

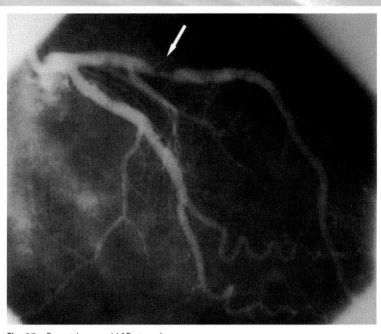

Fig. 27 Eccentric ragged LAD stenosis.

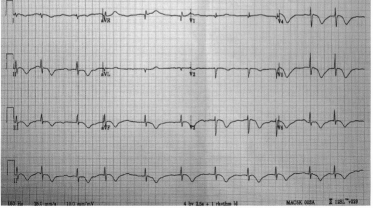

Fig. 28 Widespread T wave inversion in a patient with acute coronary syndrome.

5 Variant/Prinzmetal's angina

Definition

This rare condition is characterized by anginal pain occurring unpredictably at rest and often occurring at night.

Patho-physiology

Increased tone in focal segments of a coronary artery (coronary vasoconstriction) leads to reduction in flow. The mechanism of vasospasm is not entirely clear but it may be associated with vasospasm elsewhere, e.g. Raynaud's phenomenon. It may however complicate coronary atherosclerosis producing a mixed picture with exercise-induced angina combined with some unpredictability in the precipitation of symptoms.

Investigations

Electrocardiography   ECG manifestations were first described by Prinzmetal. During episodes of chest pain there is ST elevation (ST depression usually occurs with typical angina) returning to baseline as symptoms abate. Episodes of ischaemia may provoke ventricular arrhythmias, often with a polymorphic pattern. ST segment change may occur in the absence of symptoms, as revealed by ambulatory ST segment monitoring.

Coronary arteriography   This may reveal normal coronary arteries with no evidence of obstructive disease. Coronary vasoconstriction (spasm) may be precipitated by the injection of e.g. ergonovine directly into the coronary artery.

Management

The condition is relatively unusual and optimal management is not established. The most common approach is to use coronary vasodilator agents especially calcium channel blockers or nitrates often in high doses. Beta-blockers, in general, have adverse effects in the condition. In the presence of co-existing coronary narrowing, revascularization may be necessary.

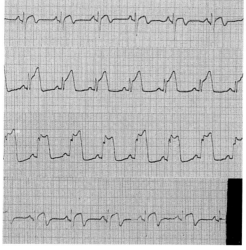

Fig. 29 ECG recorded in patient at rest showing periods of ST segment elevation associated with chest pain.

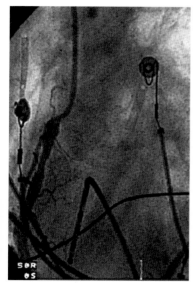

Fig. 30 Minor RCA stenosis.

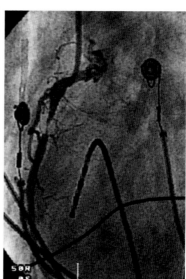

Fig. 31 Following injection of ergonovine the stenosis becomes critical.

6 ST elevation myocardial infarction (STEMI)

Incidence

Approximately 240 000 myocardial infarctions occur each year in the UK with the risk being approximately 1% per annum for males past middle age. Primary care practitioners see on average two or three myocardial infarctions per year. Early recognition is required as 50% of all deaths occur within an hour of the onset of symptoms and this can be reduced with proper management.

Pathology

Myocardial infarction is defined as myocardial necrosis following cessation of blood supply. The most common (>99%) cause of myocardial infarction is rupture or ulceration of an atheromatous plaque leading to localized thrombosis and coronary occlusion. Infarction is usually regional following the occlusion of a single coronary artery. Two patterns are described where either the full thickness of the myocardium is involved (STEMI) or necrosis is more localized to the sub-endocardium (NSTEMI). Histological changes in the myocardium are apparent only 3 hours after coronary occlusion, which explains the effort that has gone into designing strategies to reopen occluded arteries.

Diagnosis

The World Health Organization criteria for the diagnosis of acute myocardial infarction requires two of the following: typical history, ECG changes and rise in cardiac enzymes.

History   A typical history is available from the majority of patients with crushing retrosternal chest pain associated with shortness of breath, sweating, nausea and vomiting. The pain may radiate to the jaw and arms and typically builds up over several minutes. Symptoms in older patients may be atypical and not immediately referable to the heart; for example myocardial infarction may present as an acute confusional state. Under such conditions retrospective recognition is often all that is available and myocardial infarction is described as silent in 20–30% of patients. It is very important to exclude other conditions, e.g. dissecting aneurysm, peptic ulceration etc. from the differential diagnosis especially if thrombolysis is to be administered.

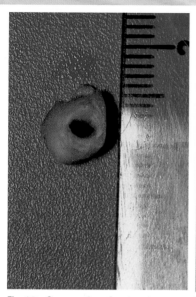

Fig. 32 Cross-section of postmortem specimen of the LAD showing the cause of MI – intraluminal thrombus.

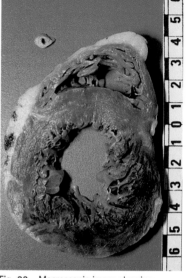

Fig. 33 Macroscopic image showing extensive transmural MI with haemorrhage and necrosis.

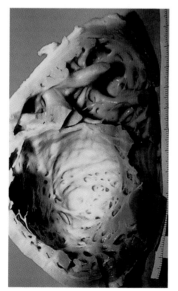

Fig. 34 Left ventricular aneurysm following full thickness myocardial infarction.

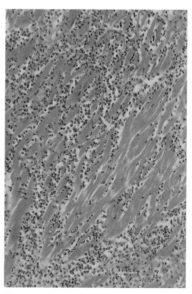

Fig. 35 Neutrophilic infiltrate in the myocardium in acute MI.

Investigations

Electrocardiography   The characteristic progressive changes in the ECG involve T-wave changes (peaked or inverted) then ST segment elevation (>1 mm in the limb leads or >2 mm in the precordial leads) all within a short time of onset. Reciprocal ST depression may be seen in the leads opposite the anatomical infarction. T-wave inversion and finally pathological Q wave formation (>25% the amplitude of the corresponding R wave) occurs from hours to days post myocardial infarction. However, a typical sequence may not occur in up to one-third of cases (e.g. new left bundle branch block). In approximately 10% of cases the ECG may remain unchanged.

Enzymes   Serial blood samples for enzyme estimation are taken to confirm the diagnosis of acute myocardial infarction, as well as to help in estimating the size of the infarcted territory. Creatinine kinase (CK) is abnormally elevated within 4–6 h of the onset of infarction and usually reaches peak concentrations at 24 h. CK is also found in skeletal muscle and can be significantly elevated in a number of non-cardiac conditions (diabetes, statin use, exercise). Cardiac troponins (TnT/TnI) have greater sensitivity and specificity than CK and are therefore useful either in conjunction with or independently of CK.

Further investigation

Plasma lipids   Myocardial infarction is often the first manifestation of coronary heart disease and blood obtained from the patient should be sent for lipid analysis. The results should, however, be interpreted with caution as the stress of myocardial infarction will influence measured values.

Echocardiography   The region of infarction may appear poorly contractile or immobile on transthoracic echocardiography. Although not necessary in uncomplicated cases, this investigation is vital in suspected acute valvular disruption or, for example, if there could be right ventricular involvement.

Right heart catheterization   Invasive monitoring of right heart pressures and pulmonary capillary wedge pressure (an index of the left heart filling pressures) by insertion of a Swan–Ganz catheter is not required in uncomplicated myocardial infarction. However, in patients with complications, e.g. shock, such information may very occasionally be considered useful, although there is a risk of cardiac perforation.

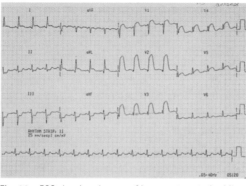

Fig. 36   ECG showing changes of hyperacute anterior MI.

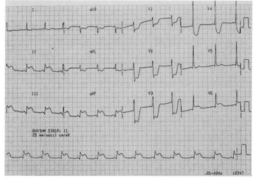

Fig. 37   Early change inferior and posterior MI.

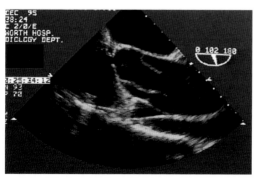

Fig. 38   Transoesophageal echo of acute aortic dissection.

Management

General

It is now recognized that an important determinant in the outcome of myocardial infarction is speed of diagnosis and management. The incidence of ventricular arrhythmias is highest during the early phases of a myocardial infarction. Consequently, all front line ambulances in the UK are equipped with defibrillators and aim to arrive within 8 minutes of the emergency call. Analgesia, oxygen and aspirin are often administered before the patient reaches the hospital. Several large-scale clinical studies have conclusively shown that early administration of an intravenous thrombolytic agent improves prognosis. Initiatives have been introduced in many European countries with the aim of reducing the time from calling for professional help to receiving thrombolysis ('call to needle time') to within 60 minutes.

Medical

Aspirin   Should be given immediately provided there are no contraindications. A 300 mg tablet is chewed then swallowed.

Thrombolysis   It is estimated that 50 000 patients receive thrombolysis out of 240 000 confirmed STEMI in England and Wales each year, indicating gross underuse. Several agents are available, all of which promote clot lysis. Streptokinase is the oldest agent and is commonly used for inferior infarcts. Streptokinase should not be given if it has already been received within the preceding year as anti-streptokinase antibodies reduce the effectiveness of the drug and may lead to allergic reaction. Alteplase, reteplase and tenecteplase comprise the remainder of commonly used agents. They can be conveniently administered as bolus doses rather than infusions and have greater recanalization rates, although at the cost of a marginal increase in the risk of bleeding. These drugs are used for patients with anterior infarcts. The maximum benefit with thrombolysis is seen when given within 6 h after the onset of pain; there is little to gain once more than 12 h have elapsed.

Contraindications to thrombolysis   Include patients with a recent history of haemorrhagic stroke, peptic ulceration or recent gastrointestinal surgery, a bleeding diathesis, severe hypertension or during pregnancy. Proliferative diabetic retinopathy is only a relative contraindication. The major complication is bleeding. Gastrointestinal and intracranial haemorrhage, occur in 0.5–1% of cases. As currently used, the benefits of thrombolytic therapy far outweigh these potential risks.

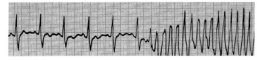

Fig. 39 Rhythm strip showing sinus rhythm degenerating to ventricular tachycardia.

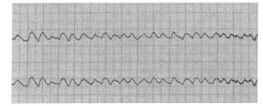

Fig. 40 Ventricular fibrillation.

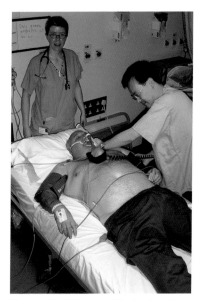

Fig. 41 Defibrillator paddles in place for cardioversion.

Management (cont'd)

Beta-blockers   Have been shown to reduce mortality in STEMI, by reducing the incidence of cardiac rupture and ventricular fibrillation, particularly in the over-65 age group. The addition of beta-blockade to thrombolysis is thought to convey additional benefit. Provided the patient is not asthmatic and does not suffer from heart failure or conduction tissue disease, a beta-blocker should be administered IV as soon as possible after the onset of infarction.

ACE inhibitors   Are thought to improve outcome in STEMI by preventing or reducing unfavourable cardiac remodelling.

Insulin   Previously known diabetics (both types I and II) and patients with abnormally high plasma glucose levels are seen to benefit from aggressive glycaemic control with intravenous insulin.

Statins   Early, aggressive control of elevated cholesterol has a marked positive effect on long-term survival.

Coronary angiography
There is no role for routine angiography following myocardial infarction. Early or 'rescue' PCI is reserved for those with ongoing symptoms without ECG evidence of recanalization, or impending cardiogenic shock. Primary PCI (angioplasty without antecedent thrombolysis) has been shown to improve coronary artery patency, LV function and mortality and is an ideal which may be difficult to deliver.

Prognosis

There are three major determinants of survival following STEMI: residual left ventricular function, extent of the underlying coronary disease and degree of electrical instability. Most patients undergo non-invasive testing prior to discharge, usually an exercise stress test on the fifth day. Those with a positive test and those with NSTEMI usually undergo coronary angiography. A low ejection fraction (<30%) identifies those at high risk of sudden cardiac death. Recent studies show that survival is improved in this group with the use of implantable cardioverter defibrillators (ICDs). The use of these devices as a primary prevention tool for sudden death in this group is likely to expand substantially.

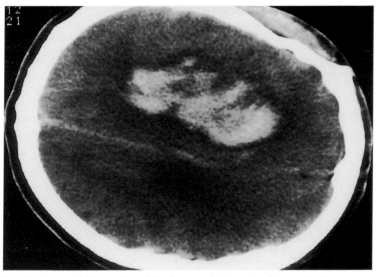

Fig. 42 Intracranial haemorrhage following the administration of tissue plasminogen activator (t-PA).

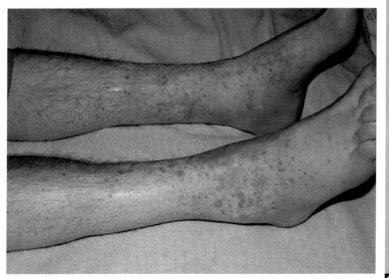

Fig. 43 Leukocytoclastic vasculitis following the administration of streptokinase.

Arrhythmias

Most arrhythmias can complicate STEMI. Ventricular extrasystoles are very common (>90%) and in general do not require treatment. Reperfusion following thrombolysis may lead to transient bradycardia which is treated conservatively. Ventricular tachyarrhythmias usually require immediate intervention, particularly if there is haemodynamic deterioration. Complete heart block associated with inferior myocardial infarction is usually transient and does not always require temporary pacing. Complete heart block with anterior myocardial infarction is associated with large infarcts and poor prognosis. Permanent pacing may be required.

Mechanical complications

The presentation of mechanical complications of acute myocardial infarction is usually with circulatory collapse and pulmonary oedema.

Cardiogenic shock   Associated with extensive STEMI (>40% of LV mass involved). The incidence remains around 5% and mortality >75%. Rescue PCI, intra-aortic balloon counterpulsation and dual chamber pacing (with complete heart block) may help.

Ventricular septal defect/acute mitral regurgitation Suggested by a new systolic murmur in a shocked patient. Diagnosis is made with echocardiography and Doppler. Surgical repair offers the only real chance of survival but mortality remains around 50%.

Ventricular free wall rupture   Causes 10% of in-hospital deaths following myocardial infarction. Incidence is reduced by the early administration of intravenous beta-blockers. Mortality approaches 100%.

Pericarditis   Dressler's syndrome (fever, pericarditis, raised ESR) may appear 2–10 weeks following myocardial infarction.

Left ventricular aneurysm   Develops in up to 10% of patients surviving myocardial infarction. Aneurysmectomy may be required.

Left ventricular thrombus   Detected by echocardiography (20–40% of anterior infarcts). Embolism may cause stroke or peripheral arterial occlusion.

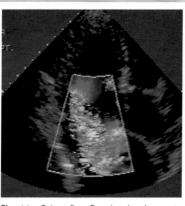

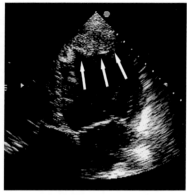

Fig. 44 Colour flow Doppler showing acute mitral regurgitation with jet demonstrated from the LV to the left atrium.

Fig. 45 Apical left ventricular thrombus.

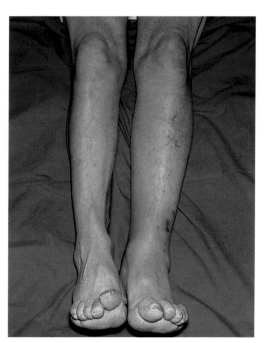

Fig. 46 Prolonged immobility following MI may lead to venous thrombosis with the risk of pulmonary embolism.

Definition

Acute heart failure is a sudden decline in left ventricular function usually resulting in both high filling pressures and a low cardiac output. In most patients a vicious circle of events is established where a decline in cardiac function leads to pulmonary oedema with hypoxia and hypotension, both of which cause a fall in myocardial perfusion and further deterioration in cardiac pumping ability.

Aetiology

Acute heart failure usually results from acute myocardial infarction and such patients will have extensive left ventricular damage and a poor prognosis, with the rare exception of surgically correctable acute mechanical complications. In patients with chronic left ventricular disease an arrhythmia or other circulatory stress (e.g. infection, anaemia, pulmonary embolus, thyrotoxicosis) may precipitate acute heart failure. Myocarditis may present with severe heart failure and a fatal course. The diagnosis of pericardial effusion with tamponade should always be considered in patients presenting with this clinical picture, since it is readily treatable by pericardial drainage.

Presentation

An acute onset of shortness of breath leads to patient discomfort and restlessness. Chest pain and palpitation may accompany dyspnoea and provide a useful clue to the underlying mechanism. The clinical appearance is characteristic with the patient sitting upright and using accessory muscles of respiration. The skin is pale, cool and moist. Consciousness may be impaired.

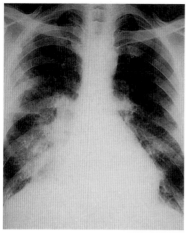

Fig. 47 Mitral valve rupture following MI showing pulmonary oedema.

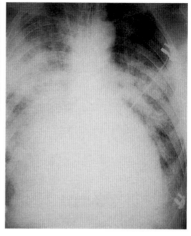

Fig. 48 Same patient as in Fig. 45 showing extent of deterioration 4 hours later.

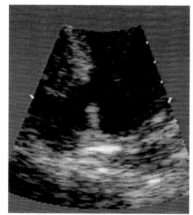

Fig. 49 Ventricular septal defect on two-dimensional echo.

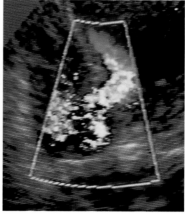

Fig. 50 Colour flow across defect.

Examination

The patient is usually tachycardic and hypotensive. The extremities are cool because of intense vasoconstriction. The jugular venous pressure may be raised and additional heart sounds may be audible. Murmurs may represent long-standing valvular dysfunction or new mechanical failure. Coarse crackles may be heard in the chest with pulmonary oedema but many other respiratory conditions can mimic this finding. Oligo/anuria is a common finding.

Investigations

Chest X-ray   Usually shows changes of pulmonary oedema, with fluid within the fissures and septal lines (Kerley B lines). The vascular shadows may suggest upper lobe blood diversion and the heart may be enlarged. A globular heart silhouette may represent a pericardial effusion.

Electrocardiogram   May reveal changes of acute ischaemia, infarction or arrhythmia. Small complexes or electrical alternans (alternate small and large voltage deflections) are seen in large pericardial collections.

Echocardiogram   An echocardiogram may help to diagnose acute valvular dysfunction and septal defects and exclude pericardial effusion. Left ventricular systolic function can be estimated.

Haemodynamic monitoring   Patients not responding rapidly to treatment may benefit from invasive monitoring. An arterial (radial) line to monitor systemic arterial pressure is useful. Pulmonary artery catheters such as the Swan–Ganz balloon flotation catheter can be used to measure right-sided filling pressures, although benefits may be marginal.

Management

Sitting the patient upright allows greater apical gas exchange in pulmonary oedema. Oxygen should be administered via facemask, with additional continuous positive airway pressure (CPAP) if required to achieve adequate oxygenation. Intravenous diamorphine relieves pain and distress and reduces preload via systemic venodilation. Further reduction in preload can be achieved with intravenous furosemide (venodilator action, rather than diuretic function is responsible for the rapid symptom relief) and intravenous nitrates. Further treatment includes inotropic support, intra-aortic balloon counter-pulsation, revascularization or other directed surgery depending on the underlying cause.

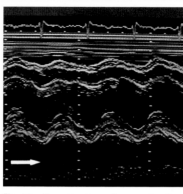

Fig. 51 M-mode echocardiogram showing large pericardial effusion (echo-free space around heart).

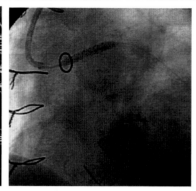

Fig. 52 Acute revascularization using PTCA in patient with cardiogenic shock due to acute vein graft occlusion.

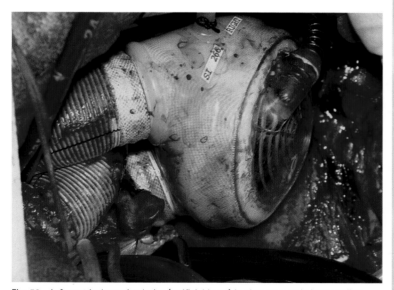

Fig. 53 Left ventricular assist device (artificial heart) in place as a prelude to cardiac transplantation.

Definition

Heart failure is present when cardiac pumping ability is insufficient for the metabolic needs of the organs and tissue. It is not a diagnosis but a complex of symptoms with evidence of ventricular disease and a specific aetiology should be established. The prevalence in Europe is around 0.45% overall, rising to 3% in elderly patients. 10% of people over the age of 75 are thought to have heart failure.

Aetiology

Coronary heart disease Is responsible for 50–75% of cases, usually in the form of STEMI-induced left ventricular damage. Some patients with severe coronary artery disease and no evidence of previous myocardial infarction may have ventricular dysfunction that is improved by revascularization (hibernating myocardium).

Dilated cardiomyopathy Accounts for the majority of the remainder (20–30% of cases).

Hypertension Is now an uncommon cause (<5%) in most European populations.

Other causes Include myocarditis, valvular heart disease, restrictive cardiomyopathy and hypertrophic cardiomyopathy (<5% in total).

Patho-physiology

Systolic heart failure The primary defect in most patients is impaired cardiac contractility. Compensatory mechanisms (such as activation of the renin–angiotensin and sympathetic nervous systems) are initially helpful but ultimately contribute to the progression of heart failure and worsening of symptoms. Therapy in chronic heart failure is currently directed to counter these compensatory effects (e.g. angiotensin and aldosterone inhibitors).

Diastolic heart failure The primary defect in this condition is failure of ventricular relaxation in diastole to allow adequate filling. Knowledge of the relative components of diastolic and systolic dysfunction in a particular patient is important, as this will guide therapy.

Assessment

The assessment of a patient with chronic heart failure should determine the likely aetiology, its clinical severity and plan therapy, including suitability for device therapy or surgery.

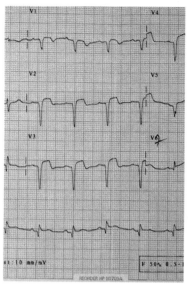

Fig. 54 ECG with Q waves in many leads indicating extensive myocardial damage.

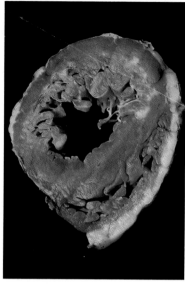

Fig. 55 Extensive old anterior myocardial infarction.

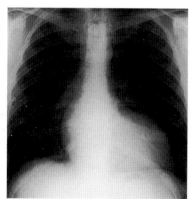

Fig. 56 Chest X-ray showing the appearances of a left ventricular aneurysm.

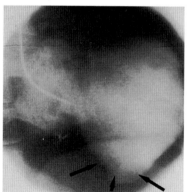

Fig. 57 Angiogram showing the same LV aneurysm as a large akinetic segment.

Assessment (cont.)

Symptoms Fluid retention leads to dyspnoea, orthopnoea and ankle swelling. Reduced cardiac output causes lethargy, reduced exercise tolerance and mental sluggishness. Symptoms may be classified by the New York Heart Association (NYHA) heart failure criteria. Class I: No limitation with ordinary physical activity. Class II: Slight limitation with activity (dyspnoea, chest pain) but normal at rest. Class III: Marked limitation with even light, ordinary activity but normal with rest. Class IV: Inability to carry out ordinary activity without discomfort, and symptoms persist with rest.

Signs Fluid retention causes a raised venous pressure, peripheral oedema, basal inspiratory crackles and occasionally ascites/palpable liver edge. Ventricular dysfunction leads to tachycardia, displacement of the apex beat and added third and fourth heart sounds. Murmurs may indicate underlying (and therefore potentially correctable) valvular disease.

Investigations

Chest X-ray For any patient with breathlessness or a raised venous pressure. The important observations in heart failure are heart size and presence or absence of pulmonary congestion or oedema. Underlying valvular or congenital heart disease may also be highlighted.

Electrocardiogram The ECG may provide important clues to the aetiology, such as evidence of previous STEMI as well as any rhythm disturbances. The presence of conduction disease (especially bundle branch block) may be important, as implantable devices e.g. cardiac resynchronization therapy may offer effective therapy.

Biochemistry/haematology Fluid retention may cause dilutional hyponatraemia. Renal impairment can occur due to chronic underperfusion in severe heart failure, which can be accompanied by anaemia. Liver function tests may also be abnormal due to chronic congestion.

Echocardiography All patients with heart failure require an echocardiogram to assess left ventricular function and exclude a potentially surgically correctable cause.

Nuclear ventriculography This non-invasive method gives a quantitative estimate of LV function. The result is often expressed as the ejection fraction (%) and the test also allows an estimation of localized heart function. Wall motion abnormalities may be seen in coronary heart disease. Asynchronous, inefficient movement of the two ventricles can occur with disordered ventricular conduction

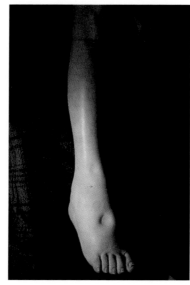

Fig. 58 Pitting oedema.

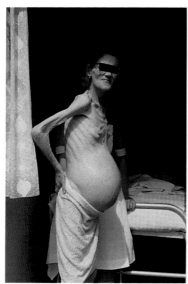

Fig. 59 Ascites associated with severe heart failure and tricuspid regurgitation.

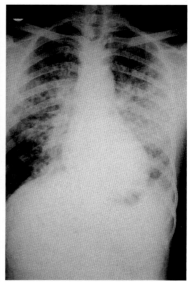

Fig. 60 Pulmonary oedema with normal heart size.

Investigations (cont.)

(e.g. bundle branch block). The presence of a LV aneurysm may be detected and suggest possible benefit from surgery.

Myocardial perfusion imaging   Some patients with coronary disease may benefit from revascularization, if imaging studies, e.g. cardiac magnetic resonance imaging (MRI), positron emission tomography (PET), demonstrate viable (hibernating) myocardium.

Medical management

The principal aims of treatment are to control symptoms and to improve survival. Patients with symptoms on mild exertion or at rest (NYHA class III–IV) may have an annual mortality in excess of 30–40%, a figure comparable to many cancers. General advice includes moderate exercise to prevent deconditioning, stopping of smoking and reduction in alcohol/salt intake.

Diuretics   Initial therapy is with a diuretic in most patients. They improve symptoms but have no prognostic benefit. Side effects include electrolyte imbalance, especially hyponatraemia and hypokalaemia.

Angiotensin-converting enzyme (ACE) inhibitors   Are a mainstay of therapy and improve both symptoms and prognosis. Patients with more severe heart failure derive greatest benefit. Common side effects include cough, symptomatic hypotension, electrolyte imbalance (hyperkalaemia especially important) and precipitation of acute renal failure in those with renovascular disease. Careful supervision of renal function on commencement is mandatory.

Angiotensin-II receptor antagonists   Are generally better tolerated than ACE inhibitors, also improve symptoms and may be useful as adjunctive treatment.

Beta-blockers   In many selected patients, the addition of a beta-blocker to existing standard therapy has a significant, positive effect on symptoms and survival. Patients with moderate disease (NYHA class II–III) and those post-STEMI gain the most benefit. They are believed to reverse some of the adverse effects of chronic sympathetic nerve stimulation.

Aldosterone receptor antagonists   Spironolactone, a weak, potassium-sparing diuretic, has been shown to further reduce mortality when added to existing standard therapy. The mechanism remains unclear but may involve amelioration of myocardial fibrosis.

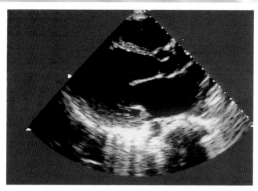

Fig. 61 Two-dimensional echocardiogram showing poor left ventricular function (diastolic frame).

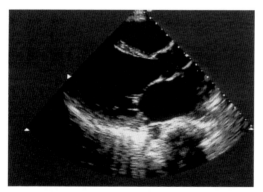

Fig. 62 Two-dimensional echocardiogram showing poor left ventricular function (systolic frame).

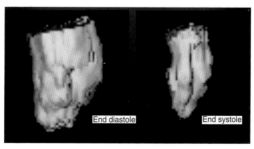

End diastole

End systole

Fig. 63 MRI three-dimensional reconstruction to assess LV function.

Device treatment

The two main prognostic indicators in heart failure are LV function and the presence of arrhythmia. Death is often sudden, with arrhythmia being the terminal event in approximately 50%. In patients with ejection fractions <30%, recipients of ICDs have improved survival both with or without previous documented ventricular arrhythmia. Abnormal intraventricular conduction is observed in up to 50% of patients with heart failure. This is recognized as a prolongation of the QRS duration >120 ms on the ECG, often with a left bundle branch pattern. Efficiency is lost with the resultant asynchronous ventricular contraction. By simultaneously pacing the right and left ventricles (via the coronary sinus), synchronous movement can be restored. Such biventricular pacing has been shown to dramatically improve symptoms and prognosis in many patients with chronic heart failure. Modern devices are now available that combine biventricular pacing with backup defibrillation and the use of such devices may become almost universal.

Cardiac transplantation

In some patients with end-stage heart failure, transplantation remains the only means of improving symptoms and prognosis. The resource is, however, limited by the size of the donor pool. Immunosuppressive treatment, usually with ciclosporin A, azathioprine and prednisolone, is required lifelong. Currently at Papworth Hospital the 1-year survival following cardiac transplantation is in excess of 90%. Deaths in the first year are usually a consequence of acute rejection and infection. After the first year survival is usually maintained for 10–12 years, after which patients tend to develop coronary occlusive disease. Left ventricular assist devices (LVADs), mechanical pumps that extract blood directly from the left ventricle with delivery to the proximal aorta, can be implanted surgically as a bridge to transplantation and indeed more chronically. Future hopes for transplantation include the use of genetically modified animal organs (xenotransplantation).

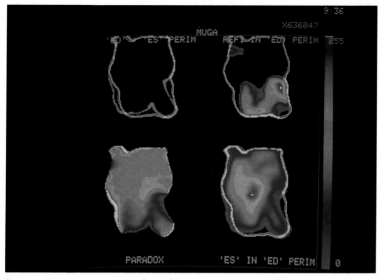

Fig. 64   Nuclear ventriculogram (MUGA) showing LV aneurysm.

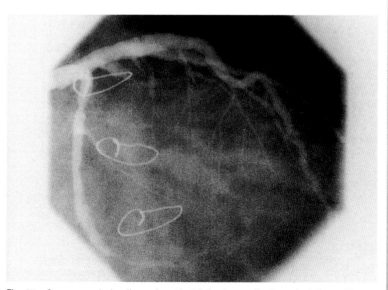

Fig. 65   Coronary occlusive disease in patient following cardiac transplantation, with tapered vessels and absent side branches.

9 Dilated cardiomyopathy

Definition

Defined as left ventricular dilatation with systolic dysfunction in the absence of coronary, valvular or hypertensive heart disease. Incidence is 5–8:100 000 with a male preponderance.

Aetiology

The precise aetiology remains unknown in most patients, despite the fact that almost 100 different disorders are associated with the condition. Genetic factors are increasingly recognized and probably account for more than 30% of cases, with familial transmission via autosomal or X-linked mechanisms. Other cases are the consequence of viral myocarditis, which may be subclinical. Coxsackie virus has long been associated with cardiomyopathy but HIV is increasingly recognized and carries a poor prognosis. Other specific causes include nutritional deficiencies (thiamine, selenium), cytotoxins (doxorubicin, cobalt), infiltrative condition (sarcoidosis, haemochromatosis), thyroid disease, and excess alcohol. Peripartum cardiomyopathy is uncommon but is usually associated with a better prognosis.

Investigations

Electrocardiography Non-specific repolarization changes, bundle branch block and atrial and ventricular arrhythmias.

Chest X-ray Cardiomegaly is usually present. Pulmonary oedema is also seen.

Echocardiography Characteristic features are of a poorly functioning dilated left ventricle in the absence of regional wall motion abnormalities.

Cardiac catheterization Useful to exclude underlying coronary artery disease. Endomyocardial biopsy is occasionally performed.

Management

As for heart failure. Prognostic benefits however have only been seen with beta-blockers, ACE inhibitors and ICDs. Anticoagulation protects against systemic embolism. Cardiac transplantation may be necessary.

Prognosis

50% mortality in the first 2 years following diagnosis but with 25% of patients surviving >10 years. Increased risk is associated with reduced ejection fraction and the presence of non-sustained ventricular tachycardia on ambulatory electrocardiograms.

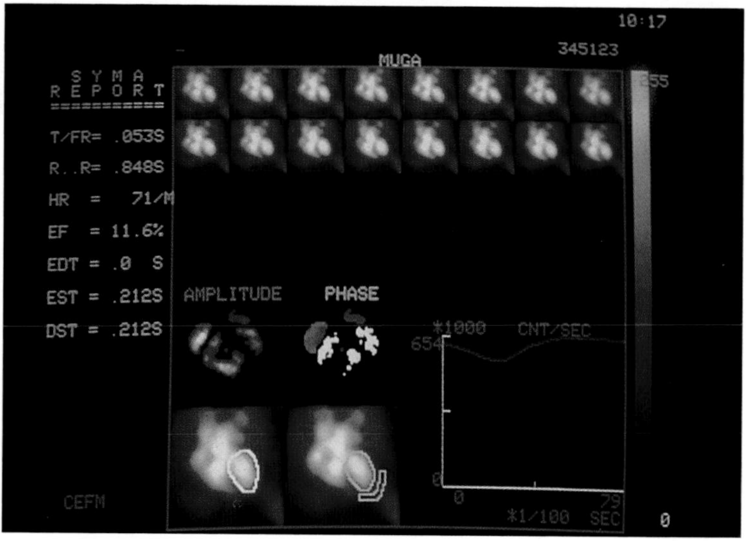

Fig. 66   Gated nuclear ventriculogram showing impaired left ventricular function (EF 11.6%) in dilated cardiomyopathy.

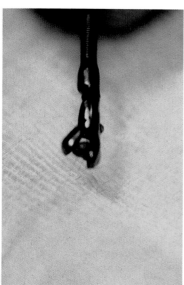

Fig. 67   Endomyocardial biopsy forceps with specimen of right ventricular myocardium.

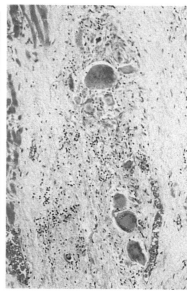

Fig. 68   Sarcoid granulomas from biopsy specimen in patient with dilated cardiomyopathy.

Myocarditis

Acute inflammatory disease of the myocardium, usually due to infection. Almost all infective agents are capable but the most common are viruses (adenovirus, Coxsackie, HIV). Non-infective causes are recognized and include drug hypersensitivity or allergy (toxic myocarditis). Clinical manifestations are variable and often subclinical. Severe cases are associated with systemic features, chest discomfort, palpitations and heart failure. Occasionally there is an acute presentation with rapidly progressive heart failure or life-threatening arrhythmia. Treatment is largely symptomatic with diuretics and ACE inhibitors. Inotropic and mechanical support (intra-aortic balloon pump/LVAD) is occasionally required. Spontaneous resolution may occur, leading to dramatic recovery, even in the most dependent patients (LVAD). Cardiac transplantation improves the outlook in selected cases. There is no reduction in mortality with immunosuppressive treatment.

Restrictive cardiomyopathy

Rare condition characterized by a thickened and poorly compliant ('stiff') left ventricle that leads to impaired diastolic filling. Systolic function is usually preserved. No specific cause is established in the majority of patients but the condition may be due to endomyocardial fibrosis, infiltration (amyloid, sarcoid) or haemochromatosis. Clinically, patients present with heart failure symptoms. The chest X-ray may reveal pulmonary congestion without cardiomegaly. The appearance can be confused with primary lung disease such as fibrosing alveolitis. The diagnosis is often first suspected at echocardiography but confirmation and differentiation from constrictive pericarditis, which has a similar clinical presentation, is difficult and important. Definitive diagnosis may need further imaging with CT or MRI, and endomyocardial biopsy. Medical therapy is difficult. Care must be taken to avoid overuse of diuretics with subsequent dehydration. Cardiac transplantation may ultimately be required.

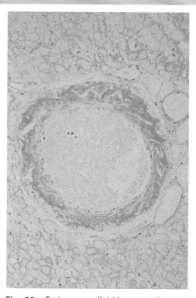

Fig. 69 Endomyocardial biopsy specimen showing amyloid (Congo red).

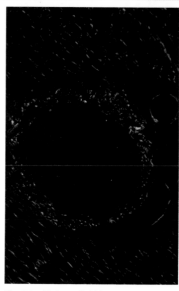

Fig. 70 Endocardial biopsy specimen showing amyloid (Congo repolarized).

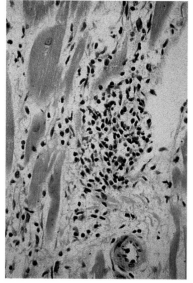

Fig. 71 Lymphocytic infiltrate of acute myocarditis.

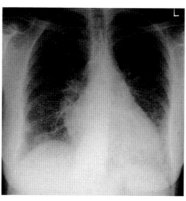

Fig. 72 Chest X-ray from patient with restrictive cardiomyopathy.

Definition

Heart muscle disease with ventricular hypertrophy (often of the septum) occurring in the absence of hypertension or aortic valve disease. Symptoms are usually due to obstruction of left ventricular outflow, impaired ventricular relaxation or arrhythmia. Affects 1:500 of the population. Many mutations have been identified in several genes. The mutations generally lead to abnormalities of structural proteins, including β-myosin heavy chain, troponin T and α tropomyosin.

Clinical features

Most patients are asymptomatic. The first presentation, therefore, may be sudden cardiac death, although this is uncommon. Breathlessness, chest pain and palpitations may also occur. Exercise often exacerbates these symptoms and may induce syncope. A large number of cases are detected incidentally on routine examination. Examination is often normal but abnormal features can include a jerky carotid upstroke, palpable atrial thrust, fourth heart sound and a variable harsh ejection systolic murmur.

Investigations

Electrocardiography   Often very abnormal with left ventricular hypertrophy, bundle branch block, large Q waves (V1–V3) and inverted T waves (V1–V3).

Echocardiogram   Diagnostic. Asymmetric hypertrophy of the ventricular septum is often seen but other distinct patterns of hypertrophy (e.g. concentric/apical) are described. Abnormal systolic anterior motion (SAM), movement of the mitral valve apparatus in systole, is a well recognized feature.

Ambulatory ECG   Non-sustained ventricular tachycardia is helpful as a predictor of risk of sudden cardiac death.

Management

Beta-blockers are used with good effect in treating symptoms, particularly those that are exacerbated by exercise, but do not reduce the risk of sudden cardiac death. Diuretics and vasodilators may have adverse symptomatic effects. In severe outflow tract obstruction, surgery, or percutaneous non-surgical septal reduction (NSSR) is an option. Implantable cardioverter defibrillators should be considered in those at risk of sudden cardiac death, but prediction of prognosis is specialized (e.g. paced electrogram fractionation analysis).

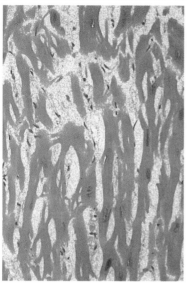

Fig. 73 Histology showing the myocyte disarray in hypertrophic cardiomyopathy.

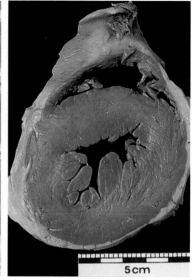

Fig. 74 Concentric hypertrophic cardiomyopathy.

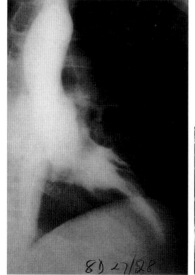

Fig. 75 Left ventricular angiogram showing characteristic appearances of hypertrophic cardiomyopathy with papillary muscle thickening.

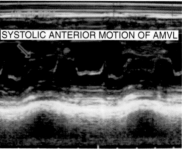

SYSTOLIC ANTERIOR MOTION OF AMVL

Fig. 76 Echocardiogram showing abnormal mitral valve movement.

12 Left ventricular hypertrophy

Aetiology

An increase in left ventricular mass in the absence of valvular disease may occur in patients with elevated blood pressure, obesity, and with physical activity (athlete's heart). Primary genetic disease (e.g. hypertrophic cardiomyopathy, Fabry's disease) should be considered but the cause may not be identified. The incidence of left ventricular hypertrophy (LVH) in the general population based on ECG recordings is in excess of 2%, but echocardiographic evidence of LVH has been found in over 10%.

Left ventricular hypertrophy in hypertension

This is an adaptive response to increased work and an adverse prognostic indicator. Hypertrophy is usually concentric with an increase in wall thickness and no increase in chamber size. ECG evidence of LVH is found in 15% of unselected patients with mild hypertension, 50% of patients with mild to moderate hypertension and 90% of patients admitted to hospital with hypertension. LVH is 10 times more prevalent in patients with blood pressure >160/95 than in the normotensive population.

Athlete's heart

The adaptive LVH that occurs with endurance training is difficult to distinguish morphologically from pathological LVH, although hypertrophy due to training often resolves on cessation of activity. LV wall thickness in excess of 1.3 cm have been found in rowers and cyclists, and ECG criteria for LVH may be present in >80% of endurance athletes. Sudden death in the setting of physiological LVH is rare. In such instances, there is usually evidence of underlying heart disease present, such as hypertrophic cardiomyopathy or coronary heart disease.

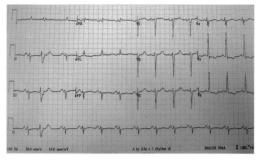

Fig. 77 ECG in LVH showing tall R waves and T-wave inversion.

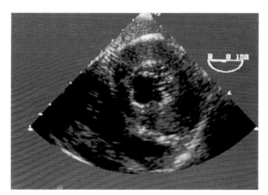

Fig. 78 Echocardiogram in LVH. Heart is seen in transverse plane with small ventricular cavity.

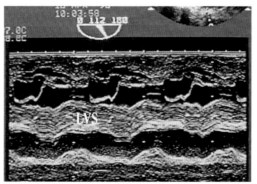

Fig. 79 M-mode echocardiogram showing severe septal hypertrophy in an athlete with hypertrophic cardiomyopathy.

IN *focus*

Clinical features	Most patients are asymptomatic. Exertional dyspnoea is the commonest symptom and is a consequence of impaired relaxation and filling of a stiff ventricle. Angina may occur even in patients without coronary heart disease, because of increased LV muscle mass and decreased coronary flow reserve. Palpitations may occur because of ventricular ectopy. Examination may reveal a sustained cardiac impulse, and an audible fourth heart sound.
Investigations	*Electrocardiography* Electrocardiography has a high sensitivity but low specificity. In the commonly used Sokolow criteria, the sum of the voltages from R wave in V_1 or V_2 and S wave in V_5 or V_6 should not exceed 35 mm; if they do, hypertrophy is likely to be present. Repolarization changes commonly accompany these changes.
	Echocardiography Echocardiography has greater specificity.
Management	Regression of LVH is seen following control of hypertension, with ACE inhibitors and calcium antagonists having significant effects. There is some evidence that regression of LVH reduces the frequency of ventricular arrhythmias but it is not clear whether this results in a reduction of the risk of sudden cardiac death.
Prognosis	The presence of LVH increases the risk of fatal events in both male and female patients with hypertension. Hypertrophy eventually leads to impairment of relaxation and heart failure may ensue. The incidence of hypertensive heart failure has decreased dramatically over recent years, probably as a consequence of improved detection and treatment of hypertension. Sudden surges in blood pressure, such as those seen in phaeochromocytoma, may still lead to acute heart failure.

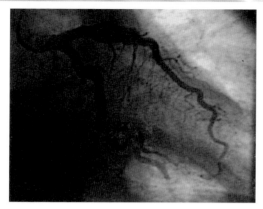

Fig. 80   Normal left coronary artery in a patient with LVH and angina.

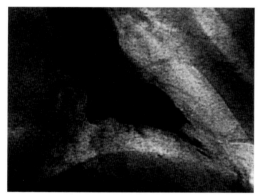

Fig. 81   Supranormal systolic function on LV angiography.

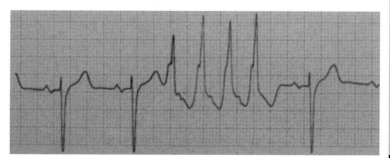

Fig. 82   Ventricular ectopy in LVH.

Aetiology

Congenital   Congenital aortic stenosis may be valvular, subvalvular or supravalvular. Valvular aortic stenosis occurs as a result of abnormality in structure or function of valve cusps. Bicuspid valves are most commonly encountered, seen in 1–2% of the general population. Valves may degenerate and calcify over time leading to aortic stenosis and/or regurgitation. Supravalvular aortic stenosis (SVAS) may occur as an isolated abnormality or be associated with a typical elfin facies, mental retardation and hypercalcaemia (William's syndrome) due to mutations in the elastin gene.

Degenerative   Calcific (degenerative) aortic stenosis is the most common symptomatic valve lesion seen in adults. Approximately 50% rise secondary to a bicuspid aortic valve.

Rheumatic   Isolated rheumatic aortic disease is now relatively rare and is usually mixed (95%) with stenotic and regurgitant components. Coexistent mitral valve disease is usual.

Clinical features

Symptoms

The three classic symptoms of aortic stenosis are angina, dyspnoea and syncope. The symptoms are often non-specific, leading to delayed diagnosis, particularly in the elderly. Angina may occur with normal coronary arteries as a result of a compensatory increase in ventricular mass. In older patients, coronary disease is frequently present.

Signs

The most important signs are a slow rising carotid arterial pulse, a sustained apical impulse and an ejection systolic murmur in the aortic area radiating to the neck but often loudest at the apex. Clinical signs can give an approximate indication of the severity of the disease but may be unreliable. Clinical assessment must be confirmed using echocardiography. Hypertension in older patients with aortic stenosis is not uncommon and the pulse pressure may be wide in view of the rigid peripheral circulation. Systolic pressures of greater than 200 mmHg are, however, unusual in patients with critical aortic stenosis.

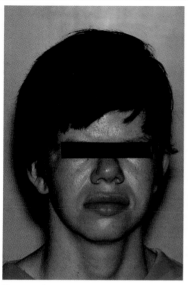

Fig. 83 Facies of supravalvar aortic stenosis.

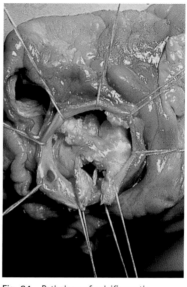

Fig. 84 Pathology of calcific aortic stenosis.

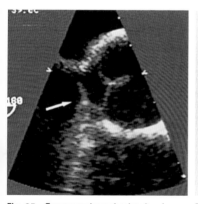

Fig. 85 Transoesophageal echo showing subvalvar aortic stenosis.

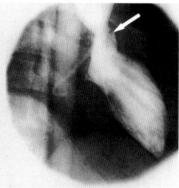

Fig. 86 LV angiogram showing supravalvar aortic stenosis.

Investigations

Electrocardiography 85% of patients with significant aortic stenosis have voltage criteria of LVH (maximum S wave V_{1-3} + maximum R wave V_{4-6} >35 mm with standard ECG calibration). ST depression and T wave inversion may later develop over the lateral chest leads (V_4–V_6), referred to as a strain pattern. Old anterior myocardial infarction may be diagnosed inappropriately because of poor anterior R wave progression. In rare patients fibrocalcific encroachment on the atrioventricular node may lead to heart block (Lev's disease).

Chest X-ray The heart size is typically normal although a bulky appearance may be suggested. The ascending aorta may be dilated proximally (post-stenotic dilatation) and is visible as a bulge at the right mediastinal border. Valve calcification is best appreciated on the lateral chest film and its absence in a patient over 35 years of age has been said to exclude significant aortic stenosis.

Echocardiography is usually diagnostic, revealing the anatomy of the valve and the extent of disruption. Doppler study allows the measurement of the gradient. LVH is demonstrated and ventricular function may also be assessed. Some patients at low risk of coronary disease (young non smokers) may proceed to valve replacement without cardiac catheterization.

Cardiac catheterization Indicated primarily in patients at risk of coronary disease in whom coronary surgery at the time of aortic valve replacement may be needed.

Natural history

Aortic stenosis typically progresses slowly and remains asymptomatic for many years. Asymptomatic individuals with mild to moderate stenosis require regular follow-up to detect evidence of progression. Valve replacement is indicated in all patients who develop symptoms and should not be delayed until irreversible ventricular damage has occurred. Aortic valvotomy (open surgery or transvenous balloon valvotomy) may be possible in young patients with congenital disease.

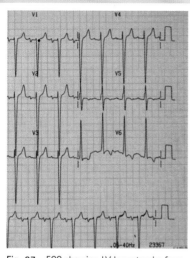

Fig. 87   ECG showing LV hypertrophy from patient with aortic stenosis.

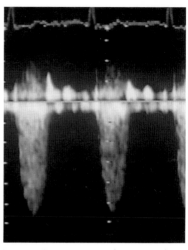

Fig. 88   Doppler gradient (>100 mmHg) across stenotic valve.

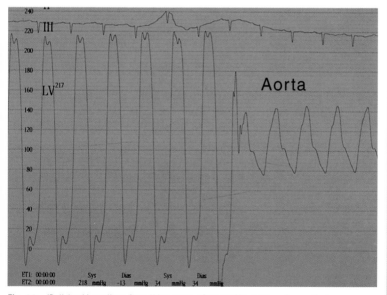

Fig. 89   'Pull-back' gradient from LV to aorta of 80 mmHg measured as catheter withdrawn across aortic valve in patient with severe aortic stenosis.

Management

Valve replacement

The significant advance in the management of patients with valve disease has been valve replacement. Valve replacement is performed via a median sternotomy on cardiopulmonary bypass. The heart is arrested using cardioplegia and the operation is carried out under hypothermia. The valve to be replaced is excised and the annulus measured, the prosthetic valve is inserted and sutured into place. Hospital mortality is usually of the order of 1–4% for elective valve replacement.

Two main types of prosthetic valves are available:

Mechanical valves   Constitute most of the valves now used (e.g. Starr–Edwards caged ball device and Björk–Shiley tilting disc).

Tissue valves   e.g. pig valves, cryo-preserved homograft, bovine pericardium.

In general, mechanical valves are resilient with a low failure rate but are thrombogenic and require lifelong anticoagulation (INR 3–4.5). Tissue valves have a limited lifespan and need replacement usually after 8–12 years. However the incidence of embolism is significantly lower and they may be used without anticoagulants, which is particularly useful in some elderly patients.

Complications of prosthetic valves:

Endocarditis   Patients with prosthetic valves need to follow recommended antibiotic prophylaxis regimens.

Embolism   The most dramatic manifestation is cerebral embolism but other vascular beds can also be affected.

Thrombosis   This leads to valve obstruction and is relatively uncommon. It can occur following discontinuation of anticoagulants. Dull thuds rather than clear clicks may be heard on auscultation and immediate surgery may be indicated.

Bleeding   This is usually a complication of anticoagulation.

Prosthetic failure   This potentially catastrophic complication is uncommon with mechanical valves (<0.1% per annum). No prosthetic sounds can be heard and cardiogenic shock progresses rapidly. Treatment is immediate surgery. Tissue-valve failure is usually less dramatic and may present with progressive stenosis or regurgitation leading to heart failure.

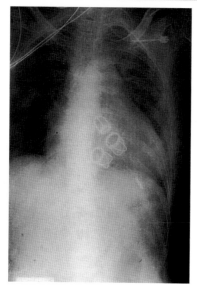

Fig. 90 Chest X-ray of three valves in situ.

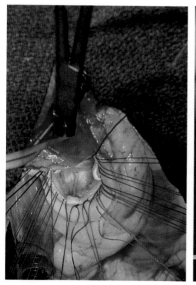

Fig. 91 Valve replacement (the operation).

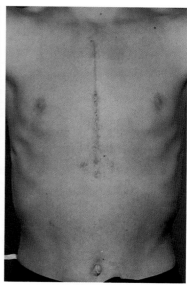

Fig. 92 Median sternotomy.

14 Aortic regurgitation

Aetiology

Regurgitation can occur because of either primary valvular dysfunction or secondary functional incompetence due to aortic root dilation.

Valvular Causes include bicuspid aortic valve (approximately 25%), infective endocarditis, myxomatous degeneration (floppy aortic valve), rheumatic heart disease (<10%) and trauma.

Root Annuloaortic ectasia, cystic medial necrosis (isolated or as part of Marfan's syndrome), osteogenesis imperfecta, syphilis and inflammatory diseases including ankylosing spondylitis, Reiter's syndrome and ulcerative colitis can be associated with dilatation of the aortic root. Aortic dissection may present with acute aortic regurgitation.

Clinical features

Symptoms
Initial symptoms in patients with chronic aortic regurgitation often relate to augmented stroke volume with complaints of a forceful heartbeat and pulsations in the neck. Symptoms of heart failure ensue as the left ventricle fails. Patients with acute aortic regurgitation, e.g. infective endocarditis, may have a very abrupt onset of left heart failure with vascular collapse.

Signs
With moderate to severe chronic aortic regurgitation the peripheral signs of increased stroke volume are usually well marked, e.g. visible pulsations in the neck (Corrigan's sign). The pulse is collapsing in quality (waterhammer). The apex beat is displaced because of left ventricular dilatation and is hyperdynamic (exaggerated normal) in quality. The early diastolic murmur is heard best at the lower left sternal edge with the patient sitting forward in held expiration. An ejection systolic murmur is almost invariable because of the augmented stroke volume. In patients with acute aortic regurgitation the clinical signs are not usually so impressive. The diagnosis needs careful consideration in any patient presenting with unexplained acute heart failure.

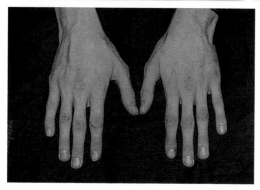

Fig. 93 Arachnodactyly (Marfan's syndrome).

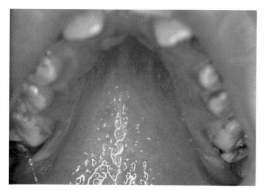

Fig. 94 High-arched palate (Marfan's syndrome).

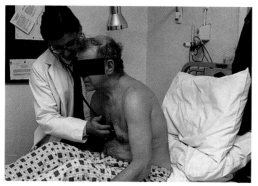

Fig. 95 Auscultation – early diastolic murmur (patient in expiration).

Investigations

Chest X-ray   Dilatation of the aortic root is usual. Left ventricular dilatation is also present and may be marked. Cardiac enlargement is not usually a feature of acute aortic regurgitation where pulmonary oedema is more commonly seen.

ECG   LVH is usual with chronic aortic regurgitation but is not a feature of acute regurgitation.

Echocardiography   Two-dimensional echocardiography is often useful in identifying the cause of aortic regurgitation. Aortic root dilatation, valvular vegetations or a bicuspid valve may be seen. Doppler studies are a sensitive indicator of aortic regurgitation and can provide an index of the severity of the disease. Echocardiography allows serial assessment of left ventricular function. Increased left ventricular systolic dimensions are an indicator of impending irreversible dysfunction.

Aortography   The classical method for defining the severity of aortic regurgitation. Dye injected into the aortic root is refluxed into the left ventricle with the volume and delay in clearance indicating the severity of regurgitation.

Natural history

Chronic aortic regurgitation is characterized by an extended asymptomatic period where compensation is maintained by dilatation and hypertrophy of the left ventricle. Approximately 50% of patients are alive at 10 years without treatment. During this phase the ejection fraction will often remain normal. Ultimately LVH and failure supervene and correct timing of valve replacement is therefore critical.

Management

Any symptomatic patient with aortic regurgitation should undergo investigation with a view to aortic valve replacement. Medical therapy may include the use of vasodilators. Optimal timing of valve replacement surgery is contentious but is certainly indicated if there is a decline in symptoms or if signs of left ventricular dysfunction are present.

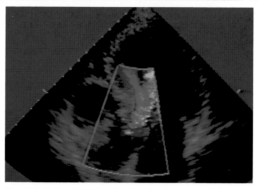

Fig. 96 Colour flow Doppler showing regurgitant jet in diastole.

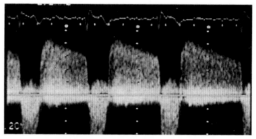

Fig. 97 Continous wave Doppler in mixed aortic valve disease.

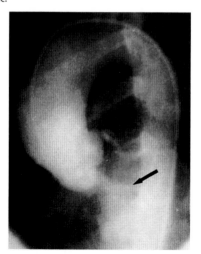

Fig. 98 Aortogram with dilation of the aortic root and aortic regurgitation.

15 Mitral regurgitation

Aetiology

Coronary heart disease   Patients with coronary heart disease usually develop mitral regurgitation as a consequence of left ventricular dilatation causing stretching of the valve ring or ischaemia causing papillary muscle dysfunction.

Mitral prolapse (see below).

Mitral annular calcification   Important cause of mitral regurgitation in elderly patients occurring secondary to the deposition of calcium in the basal portions of the mitral leaflets. Mitral regurgitation may also develop in patients with cardiomyopathy, rheumatic heart disease (usually associated with mitral stenosis), systemic lupus erythematosus (Libman–Sachs endocarditis), Marfan's syndrome, osteogenesis imperfecta and following valve destruction in endocarditis. Congenital mitral regurgitation may accompany atrial septal defects or atrioventricular septal defects.

Clinical features

The symptoms are usually those of heart failure with dyspnoea and lethargy. The characteristic finding on examination is a pansystolic murmur, often loudest at the apex with radiation to the axilla but often heard throughout the precordium. With increasing severity there is a left ventricular gallop (S3), diastolic flow murmur and systolic thrill.

Investigations

Chest X-ray   Cardiomegaly is usually present with specifically left atrial and left ventricular enlargement. Calcification of the mitral annulus may be seen. Pulmonary congestion and oedema may be present.

Electrocardiography   LVH is often present. In the patient remaining in sinus rhythm evidence of left atrial enlargement may be seen. Atrial fibrillation, however, is common. The ECG may provide a clue to aetiology, e.g. Q waves indicating prior myocardial infarction.

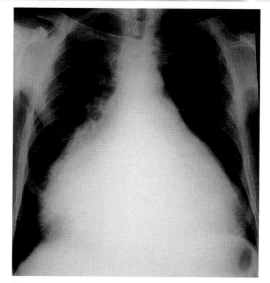

Fig. 99 'Cor-bovinum' – massive cardiomegaly.

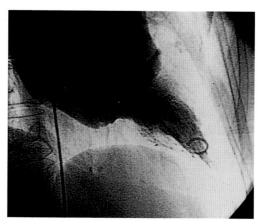

Fig. 100 Left ventricular angiogram of severe mitral regurgitation.

Investigations (cont.)

Echocardiography Two-dimensional echocardiography demonstrates an enlarged left atrium and hyperdynamic left ventricle in most patients. The aetiology may be apparent from other features, e.g. a rheumatic valve, submitral calcification, chordal rupture, vegetations, regional wall motion abnormality or flail mitral leaflets. Doppler interrogation shows a high-velocity jet in the left atrium visible in systole.

Cardiac catheterization Left atrial pressure (pulmonary capillary wedge pressure) is usually elevated with a large regurgitant systolic v wave. Left ventriculography demonstrates reflux from the left ventricle to the left atrium during systole. The rate and extent of opacification is used as an index of the severity of regurgitation.

Natural history

The natural history of mitral regurgitation is variable and dependent on the underlying cause. Timing of operation is controversial. Long-standing mitral regurgitation may lead to impairment of left ventricular function that is not reversed by mitral valve surgery. Therefore asymptomatic patients with severe mitral regurgitation may be offered surgery.

Management

Valve repair with the insertion of a prosthetic annular ring but preservation of the integral valve structure is increasingly used, although it is not suitable for some patients, who still require mitral valve replacement.

Mitral valve prolapse

An increasingly diagnosed valve lesion. Incidence dependent on the criteria applied but ranges of 3–15% are quoted for otherwise normal women. Patients are usually symptom-free but may complain of atypical chest pain and palpitations. A spectrum of disease exists from mild prolapse (click only) through mild mitral regurgitation (click + late systolic murmur) to severe mitral regurgitation (pansystolic murmur). Severe mitral regurgitation tends to occur in older males and may require valve surgery. Definitive diagnosis requires echocardiography, which demonstrates mitral leaflet prolapse in systole. Patients with murmurs require antibiotic prophylaxis against endocarditis.

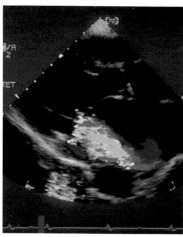

Fig. 101 Colour flow Doppler showing regurgitant jet across the mitral valve from LV to left atrium.

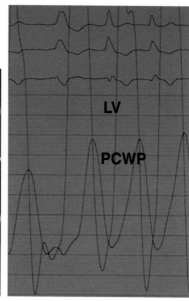

LV

PCWP

Fig. 102 Large 'v' wave in pulmonary capillary wedge pressure trace (simultaneous LV and PCWP trace).

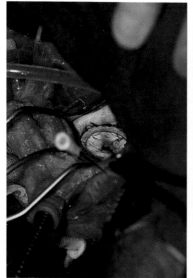

Fig. 103 Mitral valve repair with the insertion of prosthetic 'Carpentier' ring.

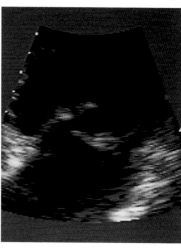

Fig. 104 Two-dimensional echocardiogram: prolapse of the posterior mitral valve leaflet.

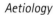
16 Mitral stenosis

Aetiology

Despite the declining incidence of rheumatic fever in the Western world, this remains the most common underlying cause. Some cases are congenital and others (very rarely) are associated with connective tissue diseases such as rheumatoid arthritis and systemic lupus erythematosus (particularly when associated with circulating antiphospholipid antibodies).

Clinical features

Symptoms

Symptoms are those of pulmonary venous congestion with dyspnoea, orthopnoea and paroxysmal nocturnal dyspnoea. Haemoptysis is not uncommon. The resultant pulmonary hypertension leads to right ventricular dilatation and right heart failure with peripheral oedema and abdominal swelling. Some patients present with systemic embolism from clot arising in the left atrium. Prior to the introduction of surgery and the use of anticoagulants, >25% of deaths were from this cause.

Signs

Patients with mitral stenosis may have the mitral facies but this appearance lacks specificity. Atrial fibrillation is common, especially with moderate to severe disease. If the valve leaflets are mobile, the first heart sound is loud and sometimes palpable (tapping apex). An opening snap is often heard shortly after the first heart sound. This is caused by the sudden tensing of the valve leaflets on opening. The closer the opening snap to the second heart sound, the more severe the stenosis. A low-pitched diastolic rumbling murmur is heard most easily at the apex with the patient in the left lateral position, in held expiration. Loss of valve pliability due to calcification is usually accompanied by a loss of the opening snap and muffling of the first heart sound. An atrial myxoma may produce very similar clinical signs.

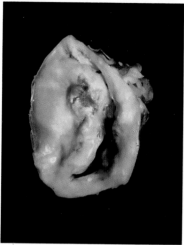

Fig. 105 Mitral stenosis with a 'fish mouth' orifice.

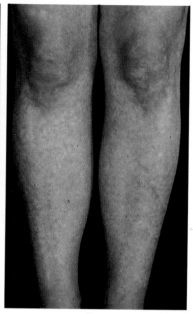

Fig. 106 Livedo reticularis in the antiphospholipid syndrome.

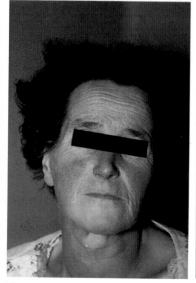

Fig. 107 Mitral facies.

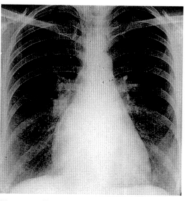

Fig. 108 Typical chest X-ray in mitral stenosis, showing straight left heart border.

| Investigations | *Chest X-ray*   Demonstrates enlargement of the left atrium and right ventricle. Pulmonary blood flow is usually redistributed to the upper lobes and Kerley B lines develop. Chronic pulmonary interstitial oedema may lead to pulmonary haemosiderosis and ossification with small islands of bone visible as dense nodules in the lung fields. |

Electrocardiogram   Most patients are in atrial fibrillation. Patients in sinus rhythm show evidence of left atrial enlargement (P mitrale). Pulmonary hypertension leads to right axis deviation.

Echocardiography   Two-dimensional echocardiography shows a deformed mitral apparatus with doming of the mitral valve and the mitral valve area may be directly planimetered. Doppler echo can assess the gradient across the valve and estimate valve area.

Cardiac catheterization   A pressure gradient is present between the left atrial (pulmonary capillary wedge pressure) and left ventricular pressure during diastole and allows calculation of the valve area.

Natural history

Symptoms do not usually develop for 20 years after rheumatic carditis, with slow development thereafter.

Management

Medical   All patients with mitral stenosis and atrial fibrillation require anticoagulation to reduce the risk of systemic embolism. Digoxin is usually required for patients with atrial fibrillation to control the ventricular rate response and diuretic treatment may also be needed.

Interventional   Indicated in symptomatic patients. Transvenous balloon valvuloplasty is the treatment of choice in most patients. With modern techniques, even non-pliable calcified valves can be successfully dilated. The technique requires puncture of the interatrial septum and inflation of a balloon across the valve.

Surgical   Open mitral valvotomy or mitral valve replacement are now needed less frequently in patients with pure mitral stenosis.

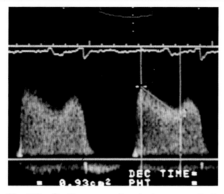

Fig. 109 Continous wave Doppler in severe mitral stenosis with valve area of 0.93 cm².

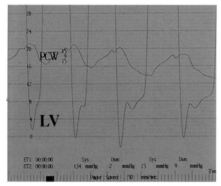

Fig. 110 Transvalvar gradient demonstrated between the LV and PWP at right and left heart catheterization.

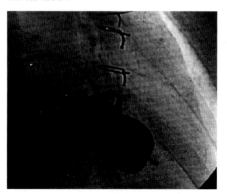

Fig. 111 Mitral valvuloplasty using the 'Inoue' balloon.

Definition

Infective endocarditis usually refers to bacterial infection of the heart valves, although any part of the endothelial surface can become infected by a variety of organisms (fungi, chlamydiae, rickettsiae, etc.).

Risk factors

Approximately 3000–4000 cases occur annually in the UK and the figure may be increasing. Patients with valvular heart disease, especially non-rheumatic (bicuspid aortic valves, mitral valve prolapse), and patients with congenital heart disease (e.g. ventricular septal defect, patent ductus arteriosus but not atrial septal defect) constitute the traditional high-risk groups. New risk groups have become prominent and include intravenous drug abusers (right-sided endocarditis more common) and those with prosthetic heart valves. Patients at risk should maintain good dental hygiene and receive antibiotic prophylaxis for dental and surgical procedures.

Pathology

Platelets and fibrin are deposited at the site of endocardial damage. This complex then becomes colonized by blood-borne organisms to form vegetations. These can grow quite large, particularly following infection with, for example, *Staphylococcus aureus* and fungi. Fragments of vegetations may embolize to distant sites, leading to infarction and/or seeding infection. Invasion into neighbouring structures can lead to valve incompetence, conduction defects and abscess formation. A wide range of organisms can cause infective endocarditis. The commonest are viridans streptococci. Specific risk groups are prone to particular infections. Elderly patients commonly culture group D streptococci, whereas intravenous drug addicts often develop right-sided staphylococcal infections.

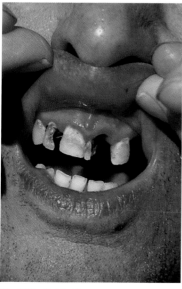

Fig. 112 Bad teeth.

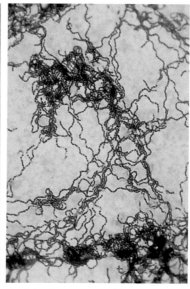

Fig. 113 *Streptococcus viridans*.

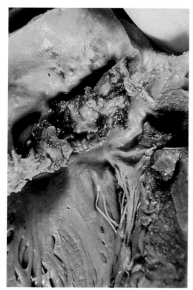

Fig. 114 Postmortem pathology of the aortic valve showing extensive vegetations.

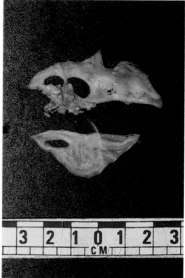

Fig. 115 Vegetations demonstrated clearly on aortic valve after removal at valve replacement.

| Clinical features | Early diagnosis is the key to successful management. Relevant features in the history include an antecedent history of cardiac disease, recent dental or surgical procedures or a history of intravenous drug abuse. The diagnosis should be considered in any patient with unexplained fever. Other common features include murmurs, splenomegaly and signs of heart failure. A range of peripheral stigmata are described that are specific for infective endocarditis. These include Osler's nodes, Janeway lesions and Roth's spots. Other non-specific stigmata include clubbing, petechiae, leukocytoclastic vasculitis and splinter haemorrhages. |

| Investigations | *Blood cultures*   Numerous sets of blood cultures should be obtained from various sites, prior to commencement of antibiotics. Blind antibiotic treatment, however, should not be delayed if there is reasonable clinical suspicion. |

Electrocardiography   The ECG is important as conduction disturbances suggest extension of the infection into neighbouring myocardium.

Urine examination   Haematuria is common. Infective endocarditis may be complicated by renal involvement (usually glomerulonephritis) and urine microscopy is indicated in all patients.

Echocardiography   Transthoracic echo allows visualization of vegetations 3 mm in diameter or greater. Transoesophageal echo is more sensitive for prosthetic valve endocarditis and aortic root abscess formation. A normal echocardiogram, however, does not exclude the diagnosis.

| Management | Mortality from infective endocarditis remains high at approximately 20%. The choice of antibiotic, the duration of therapy and overall management are best decided in conjunction with microbiologists. High-dose intravenous antibiotics remains standard practice. Valve surgery is indicated if there is haemodynamic deterioration, persistent infection, abscess formation, *S. aureus* or fungal infection, systemic emboli or large mobile vegetations. |

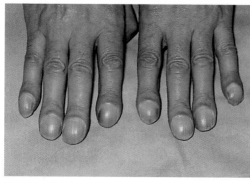

Fig. 116 Clubbing.

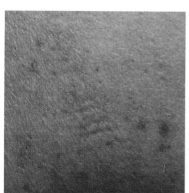

Fig. 117 Petechiae.

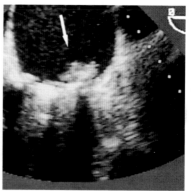

Fig. 118 Large vegetation on a mitral valve prosthesis.

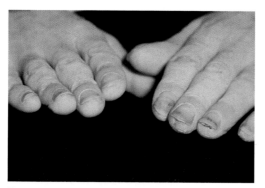

Fig. 119 Extensive splinter haemorrhages.

Acute pericarditis

Inflammation of the pericardium is commonly idiopathic or due to infection. Frequent pathogens identified include the viruses Coxsackie A & B, echovirus, adenovirus, mumps and Epstein–Barr. However, the range of aetiological triggers is wide and includes bacteria (e.g. streptococcal and staphylococcal species), rheumatic diseases, neoplasms, uraemia and myocardial infarction.

The clinical syndrome is characterized by chest pain (retrosternal, radiating to the arms and shoulders and typically eased by sitting forward) and a pericardial friction rub (scratching, scraping sound heard throughout the cardiac cycle).

Electrocardiogram abnormalities are seen in 90% of cases and typically progress through four distinct stages. Stage 1 is ST segment elevation, which is concave upwards, or 'saddle-shaped'. This pattern is seen in all the leads except V_1 and AVR. Stage 2 is resolution of the ST segment. Stage 3 is widespread T wave inversion and Stage 4 is T wave resolution. Depression of the PR interval occurs in 50% of cases and is caused by atrial inflammation. It often appears in the early stages and is regarded as a pathognomonic feature of pericarditis. The ECG changes of pericarditis can be confused with those of acute myocardial infarction. However, pericarditic changes tend to be global, have no reciprocal ST depression and are not associated with loss of R wave amplitude or Q wave formation.

The chest X-ray is often normal but echocardiography may reveal the presence of a small pericardial effusion, which may lead to tamponade in 15% of cases. Management is symptomatic with bed rest and anti-inflammatory analgesics. In most cases the disease is self-limiting. Recurrence and constrictive pericarditis are the most common complications.

Pericardial effusion

The development of an effusion in the pericardial space may occur with any inflammation of the pericardium. Effusions are often asymptomatic but, if large or rapidly collecting, an effusion may lead to raised intrapericardial pressure and cardiac tamponade (hypotension, pulsus paradoxus and an elevated JVP). Small-voltage complexes are often seen on

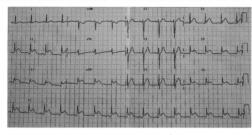

Fig. 120 Early changes of pericarditis (widespread saddle-shaped ST elevation).

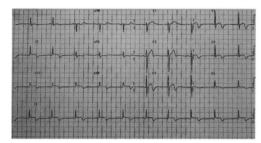

Fig. 121 Late changes in same patient (widespread T wave inversion).

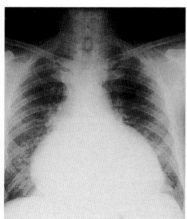

Fig. 122 Chest X-ray in patient with large pericardial effusion.

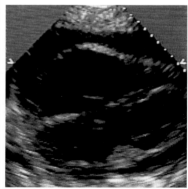

Fig. 123 Two-dimensional echocardiogram showing pericardial effusion.

the ECG. The chest X-ray often remains normal until more than 250 ml fluid has accumulated, at which point the cardiac silhouette becomes more globular. Echocardiography confirms the diagnosis. Pericardiocentesis may be required to relieve haemodynamically significant effusions or obtain material for diagnosis. Chronic pericardial effusions usually due to malignancy may require open surgical drainage, the creation of a pericardial window and in some cases pericardectomy.

Cardiac tamponade

This life-threatening condition occurs when the intrapericardial pressure rises to and above the ventricular filling pressure. The subsequent reduction in ventricular volume leads to reduced cardiac output. Any cause of pericardial fluid collection may lead to tamponade, particularly if the collection is large or accumulates rapidly without allowing time for pericardial stretch. Common causes include malignancy, pericarditis, cardiac rupture and dissecting aortic aneurysm. Clinical features include the classic Beck's triad, which consists of hypotension, elevated venous pressure and muffled, quiet heart sounds. Kussmaul's sign describes the abnormal rise of an already elevated JVP on inspiration, which may be accompanied by an inspiratory detectable (>10 mmHg) reduction of the arterial systolic pressure. Chest X-ray and ECG may be normal or display features of pericardial effusion mentioned above. Electrical alternans (alternating amplitude of ECG complexes) is a specific feature of cardiac tamponade. Echocardiography reveals pericardial effusion, with collapse of the right atrium and ventricle during diastole. In severe cases, the right heart may appear slit-like. Treatment involves the prompt reduction in intrapericardial pressure, which may be achieved with only a modest amount of fluid removed (approximately 50 ml). In emergency situations this can be performed quickly via the percutaneous route or the surgical creation of a pericardial window to facilitate drainage.

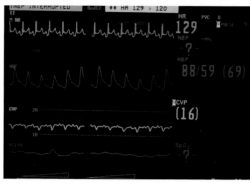

Fig. 124 Features of cardiac tamponade. Tachycardia, hypotension with pulsus paradoxus and elevated CVP.

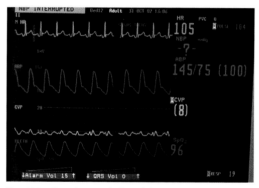

Fig. 125 Complete resolution of the above following emergency needle pericardiocentesis.

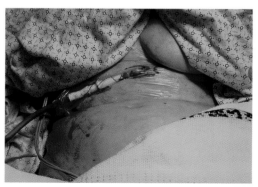

Fig. 126 Pericardial drain in situ.

19 Constrictive pericarditis

Definition	Constrictive pericarditis arises when a rigid inelastic pericardium adheres to the heart, resulting in impairment of diastolic relaxation. The common cause of constrictive pericarditis worldwide is tuberculosis, although it is an infrequent cause (<10%) in developed countries. Most cases now arise following previous cardiac surgery or mediastinal radiation, although rheumatoid disease, previous viral infection or trauma can also result in pericardial constriction. Many cases remain idiopathic.
Clinical features	Symptoms are usually those of chronic heart failure with dyspnoea and oedema. Abdominal swelling with hepatomegaly and ascites more marked than peripheral oedema may lead to a mistaken diagnosis of liver disease. The key clinical signs are raised jugular venous pressure that persists despite diuretic therapy and an early third heart sound (pericardial knock) on auscultation.
Investigations	Pericardial calcification on a lateral chest X-ray is a useful clue but is not diagnostic of constriction. Findings on echocardiography are in general non-specific. The differential diagnosis from restrictive cardiomyopathy can be difficult since they produce similar haemodynamic derangements. Differentiation depends on endomyocardial biopsy (perhaps showing amyloid infiltration) or on CT or MRI (showing thickened pericardium).
Management	Patients with constrictive pericarditis benefit from complete surgical resection of the pericardium usually carried out under cardiopulmonary bypass. Operative mortality is still as high as 5–10%, however, in most centres.

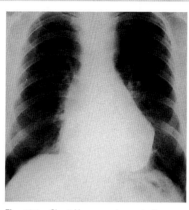

Fig. 127 Chest X-ray: posteroanterior showing pericardial calcification.

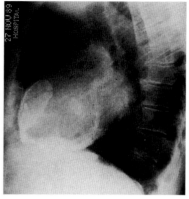

Fig. 128 Chest X-ray: lateral showing pericardial calcification.

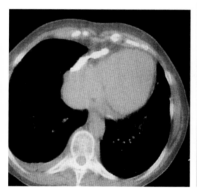

Fig. 129 CT scan: transverse cut showing localized pericardial calcification.

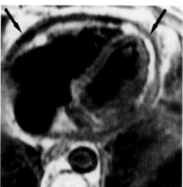

Fig. 130 MRI scan: transverse cut showing thickened pericardium as signal void.

Definition	Cardiac contractions initiated by ectopic foci, occurring earlier than would otherwise be expected. The ventricles are the most common site of origin but they may arise from the atria, junctional zone or rarely the sinus node.
Clinical features	Premature beats are one of the most common causes of palpitation. On a single 24-hour ambulatory recording, over 50% of normal individuals will have premature beats. Common descriptions include skipped beats and the heart turning over. They are usually most noticeable when the patient is at rest, particularly at night. The diagnosis may be suggested on the 12-lead ECG at the initial consultation (present on 1% of standard ECGs), but ambulatory recording may be required.
Significance	Infrequent ventricular premature beats occurring in the absence of underlying heart disease are usually of no significance. Frequency increases with age and the presence of structural heart disease. Following myocardial infarction, frequent premature contractions (>10 per hour) have negative prognostic implications. In this situation, the arrhythmia probably serves as a marker of disease severity.
Management	The majority of patients without heart disease need simple reassurance. Very symptomatic patients may benefit from drug therapy such as beta-blockade. In patients with ischaemic heart disease, especially those with myocardial infarction, suppression of ventricular premature beats has not been shown to improve prognosis and indeed some antiarrhythmic drugs may themselves increase mortality by provoking lethal arrhythmias.

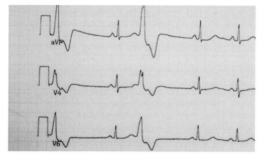

Fig. 131 Ventricular ectopy.

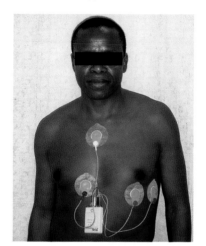

Fig. 132 Patient wearing Holter monitor.

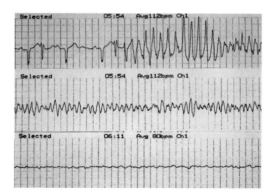

Fig. 133 Sinus rhythm leading to polymorphic VT, VF and asystole on ambulatory tape.

Incidence

Atrial fibrillation (AF) is a common arrhythmia affecting 2–5% of the population >60 years of age, but may also affect younger patients.

Definition

Characterized by rapid disorganized atrial depolarization at rates exceeding 300/min with an irregular ventricular response often at rates greater than 120/min. It is classified into *permanent* (conversion to sinus rhythm not possible), *persistent* (conversion possible with intervention) and *paroxysmal* (converts spontaneously). The main consequences are decreased cardiac efficiency and an increased incidence of stroke.

Aetiology

Most patients with AF have underlying structural heart disease (e.g. coronary, rheumatic, hypertensive heart disease). Thyrotoxicosis should be excluded in all new cases even in the absence of other evidence of the disease. Other causes include sepsis, pulmonary embolism and alcohol. Patients with no apparent cause following a careful history and exclusion of structural heart disease were formerly termed 'lone' AF. Several patterns of the arrhythmia exist. 'Vagal' AF mainly occurs at rest, often during sleep and precipitated by brief bradycardia. 'Adrenergic' AF occurs during the daytime and may be triggered by exercise. Triggering early depolarizations often arising within the pulmonary veins are thought to initiate AF in a large proportion of patients.

Clinical features

Symptoms
Recent-onset AF can cause irregular palpitations, dizziness and breathlessness. In patients with structural heart disease, a rapid ventricular response may lead to decreased cardiac output and symptoms of pulmonary congestion. Chest pain may be a feature in those with coronary disease. Syncope is uncommon, and may indicate a more serious arrhythmia.

Investigations

All patients presenting with atrial fibrillation require a number of baseline investigations.

Electrocardiography   Although a presumptive diagnosis of atrial fibrillation can often be made clinically, an ECG should be obtained in all cases.

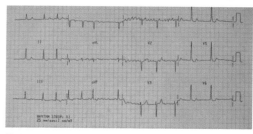

Fig. 134 ECG with slow ventricular response atrial fibrillation.

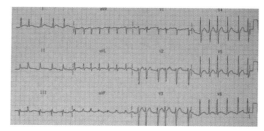

Fig. 135 ECG showing atrial fibrillation with rapid ventricular response.

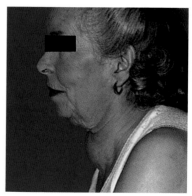

Fig. 136 Thyrotoxic goitre.

Investigations (cont.)	*Thyroid function tests* Essential in all patients, even in the absence of other thyroid signs.

Echocardiography This is essential to exclude underlying valvular heart disease, assess left ventricular function and left atrial size and look for evidence of intracardiac thrombus. |
| Complications | The main complication is cerebral embolism and stroke. Emboli may originate from the atria, the atrial appendage or the great vessels. The overall risk of stroke in patients with AF is approximately five times that of age-matched controls. In those with mitral stenosis and AF, the risk increases to 25-fold. 20% of all strokes occur in patients with non-valvular atrial fibrillation. |
| Management | Urgent DC cardioversion is the treatment of choice in the haemodynamically compromised patient. In those patients with AF of less than 48 h duration, cardioversion (electrical or chemical) can generally be undertaken without the need for prior anticoagulation with warfarin, although heparin cover is advisable. Transoesophageal echocardiography is often employed in such circumstances to exclude intracardiac thrombus. Antiarrhythmic drugs may be used to achieve chemical cardioversion in stable patients. Amiodarone and flecainide can both be effective agents. The latter should not be used in patients with ischaemic heart disease. In patients whom rate control is preferable to conversion to sinus rhythm, digoxin, beta-blockers and calcium channel antagonists are all effective. Although digoxin may provide good rate control at rest, add-on therapy with a beta-blocker or calcium channel blocker may be required for exercise-induced tachycardia. In paroxysmal AF, flecainide, sotalol and amiodarone are effective at reducing the frequency of attacks. Beta-blockers, calcium channel blockers and digoxin are of no benefit. In permanent AF, rate control with full anticoagulation (INR 2–3) is comparable if not superior to rhythm control in AF.

Non-pharmacological treatment methods are increasingly common. Catheter ablation of the pulmonary veins has high success rates in selected populations. Ablation of the AV node with concomitant pacing is effective in drug-resistant cases of permanent AF. Surgical division of the atria is occasionally undertaken. All younger patients should be referred to a specialist electrophysiologist. |

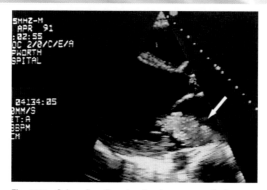

Fig. 137 Colour flow Doppler showing severe mitral regurgitation in a patient presenting with atrial fibrillation.

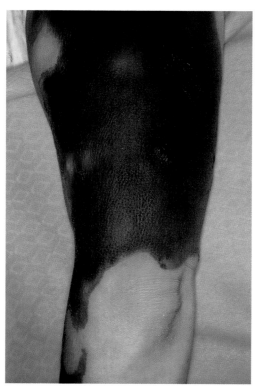

Fig. 138 Skin necrosis in patient with protein C deficiency given warfarin.

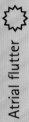

22 Atrial flutter

Aetiology

Atrial flutter is less common than atrial fibrillation, and is five times more common in men. It typically appears in paroxysmal form but persistent forms can occur, particularly in patients with corrected congenital heart disease. Although the mechanisms of fibrillation and flutter are quite different, both arrhythmias may coexist. The atrial rate of depolarization is often around 300 beats/min. Fortunately 2:1 atrioventricular block is often present, limiting the ventricular rate to 150 beats/min. Electrocardiography reveals the classical saw-tooth appearance of atrial activity, best seen in the inferior leads (II, III, aVF). Palpitations, dizziness and breathlessness are common symptoms. Syncope may occur if 1:1 conduction develops, allowing a ventricular rate of 300 beats/min. In patients with coronary disease, angina or symptoms of heart failure may supervene.

Management

DC cardioversion is usually the treatment of choice, with restoration of sinus rhythm being achievable in most patients with low-energy shocks (25–100 J). Repeated paroxysms are generally poorly controlled with antiarrhythmic agents such as flecainide and propafenone. Atrial flutter has traditionally been considered to carry less thromboembolic risk than atrial fibrillation, but current practice favours similar anticoagulation protocols. All patients with recurrent atrial flutter should be considered candidates for radiofrequency ablation.

Atrial tachycardia

A less common atrial arrhythmia (ventricular rate normally 120–220 beats/min), with unifocal or multifocal forms. Non-sustained episodes may occur in normal subjects but patients with sustained episodes usually have underlying heart disease. Incessant atrial tachycardia in childhood may lead to dilated cardiomyopathy. Symptomatic patients may benefit from antiarrhythmic drug treatment. Catheter or surgical ablation may be successful in those who prove to be drug-resistant.

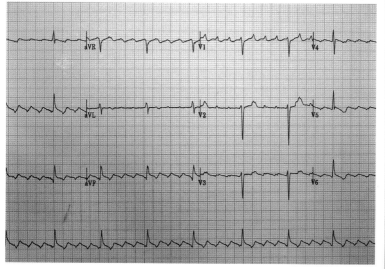

Fig. 139 Classic 'saw-tooth' appearance of ECG in atrial flutter.

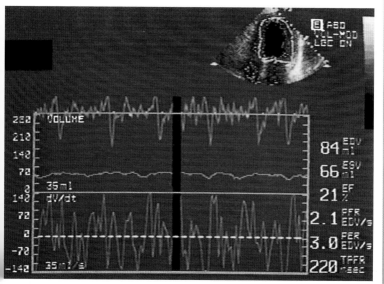

Fig. 140 Tachycardiomyopathy in patient with *incessant* atrial tachycardia.

This arrhythmia may present at any age, including childhood usually in otherwise normal hearts. It affects 3/1000 of the population, usually young, more commonly females. Approximately half of patients have abnormal conduction within the region of the atrioventricular node, giving rise to AV nodal re-entrant tachycardia (AVNRT). In the remainder, atrioventricular conduction may also occur via accessory pathways connecting the atria and ventricles, which are separate from the AV node, causing atrioventricular re-entrant tachycardia (AVRT). Circular (circus), self-perpetuating (re-entrant) conduction leads to rapid regular ventricular activation.

Clinical features

Symptoms

A history of sudden-onset rapid regular palpitation, which lasts for minutes to hours before terminating suddenly, is characteristic. Dizziness, anxiety and breathlessness are relatively common additional symptoms. In patients with pre-existing cardiac disease, angina, heart failure or syncope may be precipitated. Termination is sometimes facilitated by techniques which increase vagal tone, such as coughing, performing the Valsalva manoeuvre or taking iced water.

Diagnosis

The resting 12-lead ECG in AVNRT is normal during sinus rhythm. The diagnosis is usually obtained from ECG recordings during tachycardia. This is most commonly attained by recording an ECG in an emergency room setting and rarely by the use of 24- or 48-hour ambulatory (Holter) recordings. In patients with infrequent short attacks, self-activated recording devices may be necessary.

The typical ECG shows a narrow complex tachycardia, with a ventricular rate of 160–250 beats/min. The diagnosis may be apparent from examining the pattern of atrial activity on the 12-lead ECG during tachycardia. Abnormal deflections immediately following the R wave (P′) represent rapid retrograde atrial depolarization. However, precise diagnosis may require electrophysiological study (EPS) and curative radiofrequency ablation is performed at the same time.

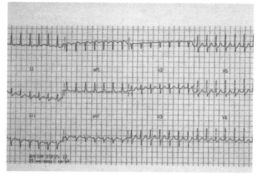

Fig. 141 ECG in patient with AVNRT.

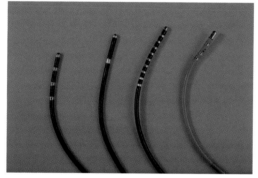

Fig. 142 Intracardiac pacing leads used for electrophysiological studies.

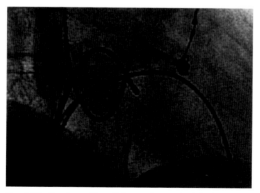

Fig. 143 Leads positioned for an electrophysiological study.

Management

Termination

Arrhythmia termination may be attempted using vagal techniques such as the Valsalva manoeuvre or carotid sinus massage. Drug termination should then be attempted using intravenous verapamil or adenosine.

Prophylaxis

The aim of drug therapy is to reduce the frequency and severity of arrhythmic episodes. Flecainide is the drug of choice for prophylaxis; beta-blockers (e.g. sotalol) are less well tolerated and verapamil is relatively ineffective.

Cure

All patients with symptomatic paroxysmal tachycardia should be referred to a specialist electrophysiologist for radiofrequency ablation.

Pre-excitation syndromes

Pre-excitation is defined as early depolarization of ventricular myocardium via an alternative route bypassing the atrioventricular node. The Wolff–Parkinson–White syndrome is the most common form, characterized anatomically by an accessory connection(s) between atrium and ventricle. Patients usually present with palpitations. The eponym refers to the ECG appearances in conjunction with symptoms; the incidence is unknown but the ECG abnormality is present in 0.3% of routine recordings. The 12-lead ECG in sinus rhythm shows a short PR interval and a delta wave (slurred onset of the QRS leading to wide complex). Symptomatic patients require radiofrequency catheter ablation of the accessory pathway.

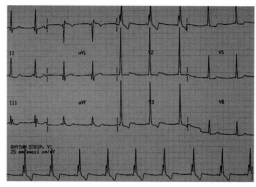

Fig. 144 Wolfe–Parkinson–White ECG showing delta waves.

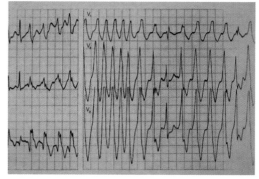

Fig. 145 Pre-excited atrial fibrillation: ventricular rate >300 bpm.

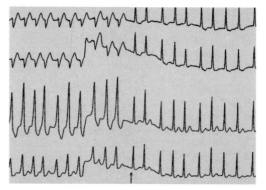

Fig. 146 Radiofrequency ablation in Wolfe–Parkinson–White syndrome: following ablation the delta wave disappears.

Definitions	Five or more ventricular premature beats occurring consecutively define ventricular tachycardia. Non-sustained ventricular tachycardia terminates spontaneously in <30 seconds. Sustained ventricular tachycardia lasts >30 seconds or requires cardioversion to terminate the arrhythmia because of haemodynamic collapse.
Aetiology	*Coronary disease* Most patients with ventricular tachycardia have underlying coronary disease and myocardial scarring from previous infarction.
	Cardiomyopathy Dilated and hypertrophic cardiomyopathy predispose to the development of ventricular arrhythmias leading to sudden cardiac death.
	Other causes include the congenital long QT syndromes and some drug-induced arrhythmias which produce polymorphic VT (*torsade de pointes*) and arrhythmogenic right ventricular cardiomyopathy (ARVC). In some patients with structurally normal hearts the site of origin is in the right ventricular outflow tract or the Purkinje fascicles and such tachycardias are amenable to radiofrequency ablation.
Clinical features	Ventricular tachycardia may produce a wide range of symptoms. It may be asymptomatic or present with bouts of palpitations, dyspnoea or chest pain; more dramatic presentations with syncope are also common. The arrhythmia may, however, be surprisingly well tolerated. Ventricular tachycardia is a bad prognostic marker in patients with coronary disease, in whom the first presentation may be sudden cardiac death.
Diagnosis	In patients presenting with tachycardia the diagnosis is usually apparent from the 12-lead ECG. Ventricular tachycardia is a broad complex tachycardia and is by far the most common cause of this ECG pattern in older patients, particularly if there is a preceding history of heart disease. Despite this, it continues to be confused with supraventricular tachycardia with aberrant conduction, where management is radically different. The principal ECG features that may distinguish ventricular tachycardia from aberrantly conducted supraventricular arrhythmia are atrioventricular dissociation, very broad QRS complexes (>140 ms) and marked axis deviation (e.g. positive QRS complex in aVR).

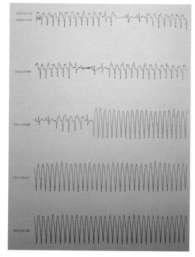

Fig. 147 Ventricular tachycardia.

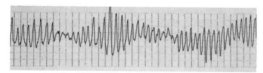

Fig. 148 Polymorphic ventricular tachycardia (torsade de pointes).

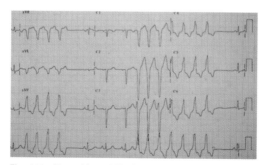

Fig. 149 Normal heart VT' arising from the right ventricular outflow tract.

Investigations

Patients with ventricular tachycardia are at increased risk of sudden cardiac death and require thorough investigation.

General   Echocardiography (with estimation of ejection fraction), stress testing and coronary arteriography should be undertaken in most patients.

Electrophysiological investigation   Patients presenting with sustained ventricular tachycardia or following resuscitation from sudden cardiac death should undergo further evaluation, which may include electrophysiological study.

Management

Management is complex and evolving and best undertaken by specialist cardiac electrophysiologists.

Pharmacological   Drug therapy aims to reduce the recurrence of arrhythmia and thus improve mortality. However, the incidence of sudden cardiac death is still significant in patients with pharmacologically suppressed arrhythmia. This situation is seen with amiodarone, the most effective antiarrhythmic drug, commonly prescribed in this situation.

Device therapy   In recent years there has been a great increase in the use of implanted devices to terminate ventricular arrhythmias. Implantable cardioverter defibrillators (ICDs) recognize the arrhythmias and terminate them via antitachycardia pacing or the delivery of a defibrillating shock. These small devices are placed subcutaneously with transvenous leads. The most recent devices have subcutaneously placed leads. Their use is likely to increase enormously.

Curative therapy   Selected patients may benefit from electrophysiologically guided therapy, with either surgery to remove the arrhythmogenic substrate or transvenous catheter ablation with radiofrequency energy. In these patients ICDs are usually also required.

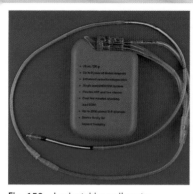

Fig. 150 Implantable cardioverter defibrillator.

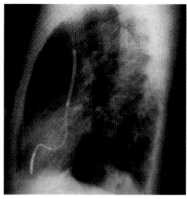

Fig. 151 Lateral chest X-ray showing implantable defibrillator lead in right ventricle.

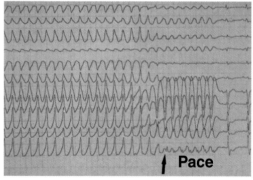

Fig. 152 Overdrive pacing of VT to sinus rhythm.

25 Sudden cardiac death

Definition	Sudden cardiac death (SCD) is defined as death within 1 hour of acute symptoms and is the mode of death in 50% of patients who die with heart disease, which corresponds to 70 000 deaths a year in the UK. Availability of effective and more widespread resuscitation has led to a greater number of survivors.
Aetiology	Coronary disease is the most common underlying structural heart defect, responsible for 65% of SCD in men and 40% in women. Patients with a low ejection fraction or history of heart failure and survivors of a cardiac arrest are at particular risk. LVH is a common finding and an independent risk factor for SCD. Hypertrophic or dilated cardiomyopathy is found in 2–3% of patients. Genetic mutations of ion channels (ion channelopathies) can lead to increased susceptibility to lethal arrhythmia, such as the long QT (LQTS) and Brugada syndromes.
Mechanism	Ventricular tachycardia or VF is estimated to be the cause in 80% of cases. Bradyarrhythmias or asystole are less common (20%). Evidence of coronary disease and healed myocardial infarction may be present, with acute infarction in only 20–25%, although this is population-dependent.
Investigations	Coronary angiography, exercise testing and perfusion imaging will together quantify the extent of coronary disease and whether inducible ischaemia is present. Holter monitoring and electrophysiological testing have a limited role in evaluating the presence of underlying arrhythmia, and their response to drug treatment. Genetic testing and family screening may be required for familial conditions.
Treatment	Revascularization may be required for patients with severe coronary disease, particularly if inducible ischaemia is present. A few patients may be candidates for surgical or catheter ablation of an arrhythmic focus. Antiarrhythmic drug treatment in general is disappointing, because of the significant risk of arrhythmia recurrence. Defibrillator therapy is associated with a low risk of SCD during follow-up and its use worldwide is increasing exponentially.

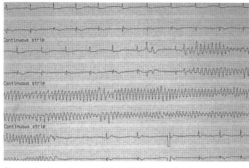

Fig. 153 Spontaneous VF on Holter monitoring.

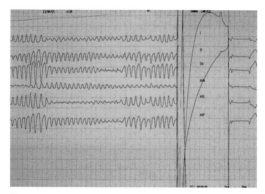

Fig. 154 ICD detects VF and delivers shock, restoring sinus rhythm.

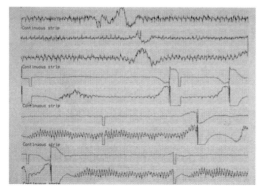

Fig. 155 Multiple shocks for VF delivered by ICD.

26 > Cardiac syncope

Definition

Sudden, transient loss of consciousness due to inadequate cerebral perfusion, secondary to cardiac dysfunction. Accounts for 1–3% of A&E attendance and 3–6% of hospital admissions.

Aetiology

Simple fainting (*vasovagal syncope*) is the most common cause.

Arrhythmia   This should be considered in all patients. Bradyarrhythmia (Stokes–Adams attack) or tachyarrhythmia (e.g. ventricular tachycardia) may present with syncope.

Postural hypotension   Often due to drug therapy in the elderly (e.g. diuretics and vasodilators) or occasionally to autonomic failure (e.g. Parkinson's disease, Shy–Drager syndrome).

Obstructive lesions   Patients with aortic stenosis, hypertrophic cardiomyopathy and pulmonary hypertension may present with syncope.

Investigations

The initial key to appropriate management is a careful history. Evidence of atrioventricular block or other conduction anomaly may be present on the resting ECG. Carotid sinus massage may reproduce symptoms and be associated with bradycardia. Ambulatory electrocardiography may reveal a specific cause such as atrioventricular block or paroxysmal tachycardia. In some patients with otherwise unexplained syncope, symptoms can be reproduced by prolonged lying with a head-up tilt, using a specifically designed table. Occasionally, electrophysiological testing may be necessary.

Management

Patients with syncope due to bradycardia detected during Holter monitoring or tilt testing may benefit from the insertion of a pacemaker. Some patients with a positive tilt test benefit from salt supplementation, advice on leg crossing and avoidance or possibly drug treatment (e.g. midodrine). In many patients, despite extensive investigations, no specific cause is identified. The outlook for survival in patients with no structural heart disease is excellent, although morbidity may remain high.

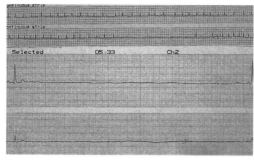

Fig. 156 Sinus node disease with prolonged pauses in patient with syncope needing pacemaker.

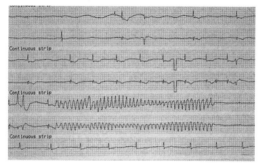

Fig. 157 Brady- and tachyarrhythmias on Holter monitoring.

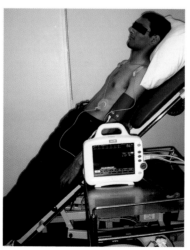

Fig. 158 Tilt table.

Pacemakers are highly cost-effective. In appropriate patients pacing cures symptoms and improves prognosis. Several million pacemakers have now been implanted worldwide but their use differs significantly between countries. In the mid 1980s use in sinoatrial disease in the USA was 8 times that of the UK. Despite a decline of 25% in the US implantation rate in the late 1980s, rates are still higher than in Europe.

Indications

Atrioventricular block   All patients with congenital complete heart block should probably be paced. Patients with acquired complete heart block (and probably those with second-degree AV block) should all receive a pacemaker whether symptomatic or not in order to improve prognosis.

Sinoatrial disease (sick sinus syndrome)   These patients should receive a pacemaker if they have symptomatic bradycardia.

Presentation

Asymptomatic   Any patient found to have complete heart block should be referred for pacemaker implantation.

Symptomatic bradycardia   Patients with a slow pulse and dizzy spells, fatigue, dyspnoea or congestive heart failure usually benefit from pacemaker implantation.

Stokes–Adams attacks   A patient with syncope and a history compatible with Stokes–Adams attack should be thoroughly investigated. Evidence of complete heart block is an absolute indication for the implantation of a permanent pacemaker.

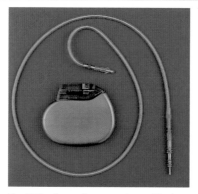

Fig. 159 Pacemaker generator and lead.

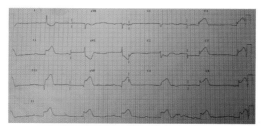

Fig. 160 Complete heart block. Atrial and ventricular activity dissociated.

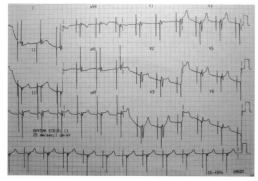

Fig. 161 ECG of dual-chamber pacemaker pacing with appropriate sensed and paced atrial and ventricular activation.

Aetiology

Conduction system disease

The majority of patients requiring a pacemaker have idiopathic degeneration of part of the cardiac conducting system. Coronary disease may be the underlying problem. In addition, some patients with combined skeletal and heart muscle disease (e.g. dystrophia myotonica) may develop heart block. Kearns–Sayre syndrome is the rare combination of progressive external ophthalmoplegia, retinal pigmentary degeneration and progressive impairment of cardiac conduction. Other causes of heart block include infiltrative disease such as sarcoidosis, rheumatoid arthritis or amyloidosis, and infections such as Lyme disease.

Procedure

The implantation is performed under local anaesthetic. The right ventricular lead of the pacemaker lead is advanced to the apex of the ventricle, and the right atrial lead is positioned within the right atrial appendage, both usually via the cephalic or subclavian veins. The pacemaker generator is then placed subcutaneously on the anterior chest wall. The patient usually remains in hospital overnight.

Pacemaker types

An international code has been established to describe available pacemaker types. The most basic type currently used is the ventricular demand unit (VVI). This relatively inexpensive device is capable of preventing major symptoms of syncope and improves prognosis. Because VVI pacemakers do not provide co-ordinated atrial and ventricular contraction or increase the pacing rate on exercise, they are not optimal therapy in most patients. Rate responsive pacemakers (AAIR, VVIR, etc.) have a sensor that increases the rate of discharge with physical activity. Dual-chamber pacemakers (DDDs) sense and pace both atrium and ventricle and provide atrioventricular co-ordination. Two pacing wires are required but they provide a more physiological replacement of the normal conducting system: the incidence of atrial fibrillation, stroke and left ventricular failure are reduced when DDDs are implanted in preference to VVI units in patients with sinus node disease.

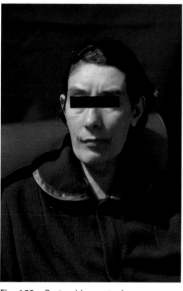

Fig. 162 Dystrophia myotonica.

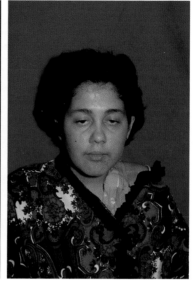

Fig. 163 Kearns–Sayre syndrome.

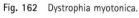

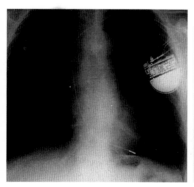

Fig. 164 VVI pacemaker (single lead).

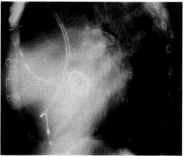

Fig. 165 DDD pacemaker (atrial and ventricular leads).

Complications

If a patient presents with unexplained symptoms following pacemaker insertion, the pacing centre responsible for that patient should be contacted.

Early complications

Lead displacement   Recurrence of the initial symptoms may be a presenting feature if primary problem is loss of capture. If the problem is a failure to sense intrinsic cardiac activity then palpitations are more usual.

Early or late complications

Myoinhibition   Some patients complain of dizziness and occasionally syncope on arm movement. Electrical signals deriving from activity of the pectoral muscles are detected by the pacemaker and identified as cardiac, leading to an inappropriate reduction of pacemaker discharge.

Infection   occurs in 1–2% of implants and presents with pain over the pacemaker site. If the system itself is infected the entire unit must be removed. Infection usually presents in the first few weeks following implantation but occasionally much later.

Thrombosis   Oedema of the arm on the side of pacemaker insertion may occur (<1% of patients) and if severe may be improved by anticoagulation.

Pacemaker syndrome   is a major disadvantage of VVI pacing. It is characterized by dizziness and heavy palpitations due to loss of properly timed atrial systole. Cure usually follows upgrade to a dual chamber system.

Late complications

Lead fracture or battery failure   Usually presents with recurrence of the initial symptoms.

Erosion   The generator or wire may erode through the overlying skin, inevitably leading to infection. Early surgery is needed to limit the spread of infection.

Superior vena cava syndrome   Rarely, patients develop stenosis of the superior vena cava with symptoms of upper body swelling and headache.

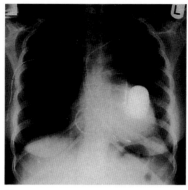

Fig. 166 Multiple pacemaker leads
following many complications and procedures.

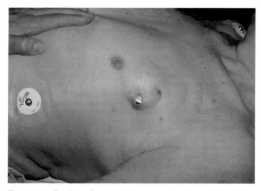

Fig. 167 Erosion of pacemaker generator through the skin.

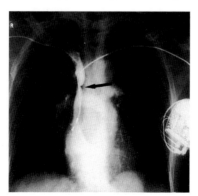

Fig. 168 SVC stenosis due to pacemaker
lead.

28 Atrial septal defect (ASD)

Incidence	The most common (30%) congenital heart abnormality detected in adult patients, despite constituting just 6% of congenital heart disease in children.
Classification	*Ostium secundum* Most common type, occurring in 70% of cases. Located in the fossa ovalis, it occurs more commonly in females (ratio 3:1) and 20–30% have associated mitral valve prolapse.
	Sinus venosus (15% of total) occurs in upper portion of the interatrial septum and is often accompanied by partial anomalous pulmonary venous drainage.
	Ostium primum Sited in the lower septum. This type most commonly presents in childhood (often in Down's syndrome) and is usually associated with other abnormalities.
Clinical features	Adults present with fatigue, dyspnoea, palpitations and chest pain. The characteristic sign is wide, fixed splitting of the second heart sound. A pulmonary flow murmur is usual and, with large shunts, a tricuspid flow murmur may be heard.
Investigations	*Chest X-ray* in uncomplicated cases reveals a small aortic knuckle and pulmonary plethora. Right-sided chambers may become dilated with time and onset of right heart failure.
	Electrocardiography Ostium secundum ASDs often have right bundle branch block, which is usually incomplete (rSr′ complex with QRS duration <0.10 s) and right axis deviation.
	Echocardiography The defect is demonstrated along with right ventricular volume overload and paradoxical septal motion.
	Right heart catheterization Demonstrates a step-up in oxygen saturation between the venae cavae and the right atrium, allowing quantification of the shunt.
Management	Operative closure is usually recommended in symptomatic patients if pulmonary to systemic blood flow ratio >1.5:1. The operation reverses haemodynamic abnormalities and reduces the potential complications of right heart failure, paradoxical embolism and pulmonary vascular disease.

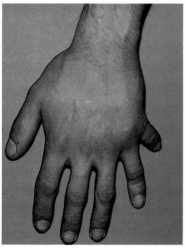

Fig. 169 Multiple digits may occur in patients with ASD.

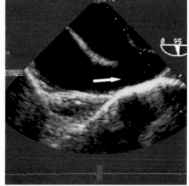

Fig. 170 Sinus venosus defect.

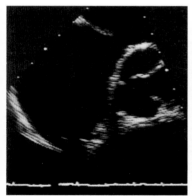

Fig. 171 Ostium secundum defect.

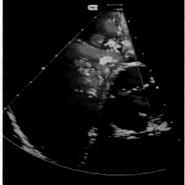

Fig. 172 Colour flow Doppler with flow across defect.

Incidence	Most common congenital heart defect (30%), although most are detected before adulthood because of prominent physical signs. In addition to occurring as a congenital abnormality, VSD may complicate acute myocardial infarction. The defect may occur anywhere along the ventricular septum but is most common in the membranous septum (70%). Seen in association with an ASD in Down's syndrome.
Clinical features	The presentation of VSD in adulthood is rare but usually follows the detection of a murmur or the development of complications. The classic murmur is harsh, pansystolic and sited at the lower left sternal edge. An accompanying thrill is usual. 5–10% have aortic regurgitation due to prolapse of a valve leaflet into the defect.
Investigations	Diagnosis is by echocardiography. Identification of small defects (*maladie de Roger*) is facilitated by colour-flow Doppler. Chest X-ray appearances are non-specific but demonstrate pulmonary plethora due to increased pulmonary blood flow.
Management	Small defects are managed expectantly, with >30% chance of spontaneous closure in young patients. Large defects with a pulmonary:systemic flow ratio of >2:1 and right ventricular overload require surgical closure. Patients are at risk of endocarditis and therefore require prophylactic antibiotics.

Fallot's tetralogy

Most common form of cyanotic congenital heart disease. Consists of pulmonary stenosis or atresia, VSD, dextroposition of the aorta over-riding the septal defect and right ventricular hypertrophy. Survival into adulthood is now common, although patients remain at considerable risk of a range of complications.

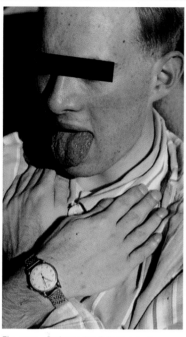

Fig. 173   Patient with Fallot's tetralogy.

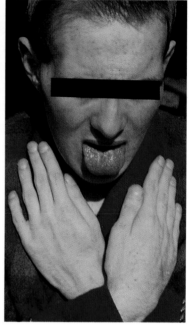

Fig. 174   Complete repair results in disappearance of cyanosis.

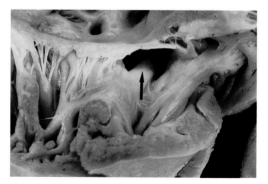

Fig. 175   Ventricular septal defect in Fallot's tetralogy.

30 Pulmonary stenosis/Peripheral pulmonic stenosis

Incidence

10–12% of congenital heart disease. Acquired pulmonary stenosis is unusual but may occur in rheumatic heart disease, following trauma and, rarely, due to the carcinoid syndrome (tricuspid stenosis with regurgitation is more common). Pulmonary stenosis may occur as part of Noonan's syndrome.

Clinical features

Usually asymptomatic but may present with dyspnoea, fatigue and, occasionally, chest pain with exertional syncope. The key physical finding is of a systolic murmur at the upper left sternal edge. An ejection click is often present and the second heart sound is soft and delayed. There is usually a thrill in the same area.

Investigations

Chest X-ray   The pulmonary artery is dilated (poststenotic dilatation) with reduced pulmonary vascular markings in severe pulmonary stenosis. The right ventricle may become grossly enlarged.

Electrocardiography   Right axis deviation, right bundle branch block and right ventricular hypertrophy are often seen.

Echocardiography   provides the diagnosis, with Doppler allowing estimation of the transvalvular gradient and hence quantification of severity.

Right heart catheterization   A gradient is observed on withdrawal across the stenosis. Right ventricular angiography shows doming of the valve.

Management

As the valve lesion tends to be non-progressive, asymptomatic patients with mild to moderate stenosis do not require treatment. Symptomatic patients with moderate or severe stenosis (gradient >60 mmHg) or with evidence of right ventricular dysfunction usually require treatment. This is now most commonly performed with transvenous balloon valvuloplasty.

Peripheral pulmonic stenosis

Some patients have supravalvular pulmonary stenosis, which may consist of multiple narrowings of primary and more peripheral branches of the pulmonary arteries. This is often seen as part of the rubella syndrome.

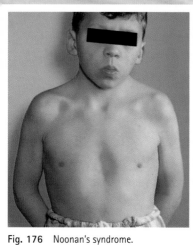

Fig. 176 Noonan's syndrome.

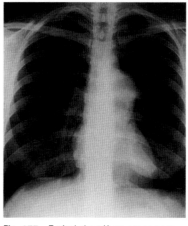

Fig. 177 Typical chest X-ray appearance.

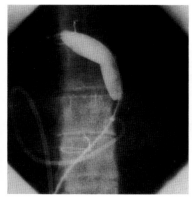

Fig. 178 Pulmonary balloon valvuloplasty.

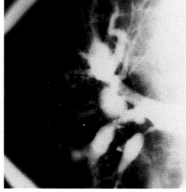

Fig. 179 Angiogram of peripheral pulmonic stenoses.

31 Coarctation of the aorta

Definition

Coarctation of the aorta is due to a localized shelf-like thickening of the aortic lumen usually opposite the ligamentum arteriosum. In adults, postductal coarctation is usual and males are affected twice as commonly as females. There is an association with Turner's syndrome and bicuspid aortic valve.

Clinical features

Most adults with coarctation are asymptomatic but may complain of headache, claudication or fatigue. Recurrent miscarriages can occur in women. Coarctation is usually detected on routine examination, with hypertension and diminished femoral pulses. Signs of bicuspid aortic valve are present in 30%. A murmur is often present over the back, due to increased collateral flow.

Investigations

Chest X-ray   Left ventricular enlargement is possible and notching on the lower posterior border of the ribs 3–8 is common. Dilatation of the aorta around the site of the narrowing may be seen.

Electrocardiography   Evidence of left ventricular hypertrophy is usually present.

Echocardiography   Not normally definitive. MRI allows visualization of the narrowed aortic segment.

Aortography   identifies the site of obstruction, demonstrates the extent of collateral filling and also allows measurement of the pressure gradient.

Management

Surgery remains the treatment of choice. Without treatment, mean life expectancy is 35 years. Death occurs as a result of the consequences of long-standing hypertension – cerebrovascular disease, left ventricular failure and aortic dissection. Subarachnoid haemorrhage is particularly common because of the increased incidence of berry aneurysm. Improvement in prognosis is achieved with surgery, although hypertension usually remains postoperatively. In one study 70% of patients were hypertensive 30 years following surgery.

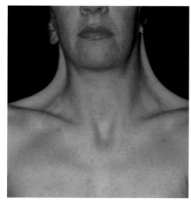

Fig. 180 Webbing of the neck in Turner's syndrome.

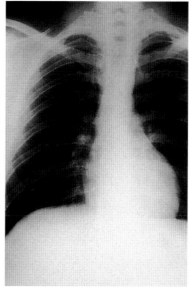

Fig. 181 Typical chest X-ray.

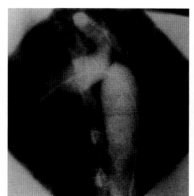

Fig. 182 Aortogram.

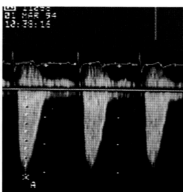

Fig. 183 Echo Doppler of coarctation with gradient of 40 mmHg.

Definition	Persistent arterial channel connecting aortic isthmus to the left pulmonary artery, now rarely seen in adults.
Presentation	The anomaly is usually asymptomatic but there is a risk of developing heart failure, shunt reversal with development of Eisenmenger's syndrome and bacterial endarteritis, any of which may bring the condition to light.
Diagnosis	Continuous (machinery) murmur is of maximal intensity in the second left intercostal interspace. Chest X-ray may show cardiac enlargement and pulmonary plethora. Calcification of the ductus may lead to a characteristic appearance in older patients.
Management	Ligation of the duct in childhood or resection in adults is curative if performed prior to development of pulmonary hypertension. Indicated in all patients to reduce the risk of complications.

Sinus of Valsalva fistula

Although rare, sinus of Valsalva fistula is the second most common cause of a continuous murmur in adults. Sinus aneurysms may be congenital or occur secondary to infective endocarditis. Rupture usually occurs into the right ventricle and is associated with an acute attack of chest pain and possibly acute heart failure. The murmur is best heard in the second right intercostal space. Colour-flow Doppler is diagnostic and the lesion can also be demonstrated by aortography. Surgical closure reduces the risk of ventricular dysfunction, infective endocarditis, septic pulmonary embolism and shunt reversal.

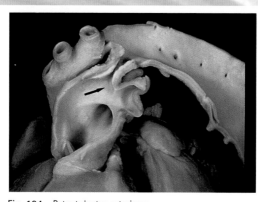

Fig. 184   Patent ductus arteriosus.

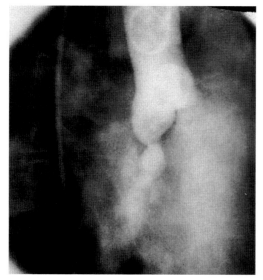

Fig. 185   Aortogram of sinus of Valsalva fistula showing flow between the right coronary sinus and the right ventricle.

33 Eisenmenger's syndrome

Definition	Eisenmenger's complex comprises a ventricular septal defect with pulmonary hypertension and right to left shunting of blood through the defect, leading to systemic desaturation. Eisenmenger's syndrome occurs following reversal of any left-to-right shunt (usually a VSD, PDA or atrioventricular septal defect and occasionally an ostium secundum ASD) following the development of pulmonary hypertension. Pulmonary hypertension develops as a result of thickening of the walls of the pulmonary arterial bed, the precise mechanism of which is not established.
Clinical features	Associated with symptoms of dyspnoea, fatigue and haemoptysis. Cyanosis and clubbing are present. The unusual appearance of differential cyanosis with blue, clubbed toes and pink lips and fingers occurs following shunt reversal through a PDA. Chest X-ray appearances may be bizarre, with a very prominent pulmonary trunk and pulmonary arteries with peripheral oligaemia. Evidence of right ventricular enlargement is often present.
Management	Individuals with cyanotic congenital heart disease, including Eisenmenger's syndrome, now commonly survive into adulthood. Long-term complications include polycythaemia (need regular venesection), gout (prophylactic allopurinol often indicated), contraceptive advice (pregnancy usually poorly tolerated) and endocarditis. Patients require lifelong specialist follow-up. Overall life expectancy is shortened. Selected patients may be candidates for heart–lung transplantation.

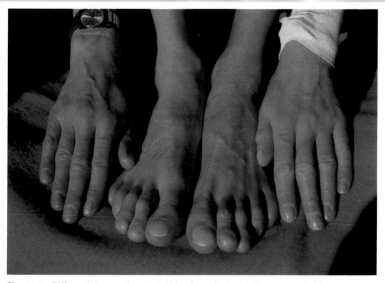

Fig. 186   Differential cyanosis and clubbing in patient with Eisenmenger's PDA.

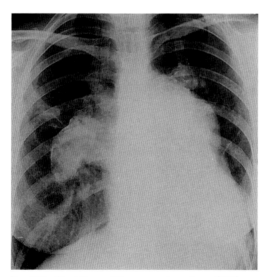

Fig. 187   Chest X-ray of Eisenmenger's syndrome (ASD).

Aetiology

Aneurysms of the thoracic aorta are relatively uncommon. There are a number of causes.

Arteriosclerosis is the most common cause and may develop in any part of the thoracic aorta. The entire aorta may be ectatic and usually there is widespread arteriosclerosis elsewhere. The aneurysm itself is usually fusiform.

Cystic medial necrosis may result in annulo-aortic ectasia and is a common component of Marfan's syndrome and Ehlers–Danlos syndrome. Aortic dissection, rupture or regurgitation may develop. Annulo-aortic ectasia is present in 5–10% of patients requiring aortic valve replacement.

Syphilis Aneurysms develop in 5–10% patients with syphilitic aortitis. Patients develop a destructive aortitis that involves both the ascending aorta and the arch. Aortic regurgitation commonly develops because of involvement of the aortic valve cusps and angina may occur as a result of coronary ostial stenosis. Aneurysms may become huge and erode the sternum and ribs. On chest X-ray, calcification is usually present in the aortic wall.

Management

Most patients are asymptomatic and come to light following a routine chest X-ray. Prophylactic surgical replacement is often needed in patients with large aneurysms, but may carry significant risks.

Aortitis

Inflammation of the wall of the aorta is termed aortitis and may occur for a host of reasons. Syphilis is a well-recognized cause but is now uncommon. Other causes include ankylosing spondylitis, Reiter's syndrome, ulcerative colitis and Takayasu's arteritis.

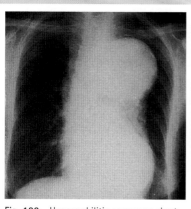

Fig. 188 Huge syphilitic aneurysm: chest X-ray.

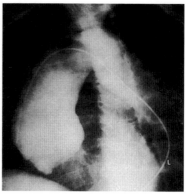

Fig. 189 An aortogram of the same aneurysm.

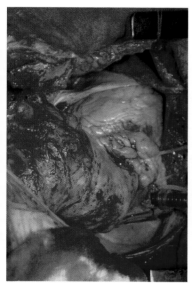

Fig. 190 The aneurysm in Fig. 185: intraoperative.

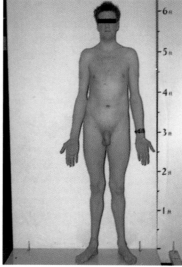

Fig. 191 Marfan's syndrome.

Aortic tear followed by tracking of blood into the aortic media. The usual site is the ascending aorta (type A) but dissection of the descending aorta (type B) also occurs. Predisposing causes include hypertension (70–90% of patients have history of hypertension), Marfan's syndrome, Ehlers–Danlos syndrome, bicuspid aortic valve and chest trauma. Males are affected more commonly than females (3:1) but dissection is described, for example, in pregnancy.

Presentation

Sudden onset of severe precordial or interscapular pain is characteristic. Blood pressure is often increased (in 50–70%) despite a shock like state. An early diastolic murmur may be present. The crucial differential diagnosis is acute myocardial infarction, as thrombolytics in dissection usually prove catastrophic.

Investigations

Chest X-ray   Abnormal in 80%, with mediastinal widening and left pleural effusion being the most common abnormalities. However, the chest X-ray may be normal.

Electrocardiogram   Usually shows LVH resulting from predisposing hypertension but there are no specific changes. It helps to exclude other causes of chest pain, particularly myocardial infarction, which may coexist with dissection (due to obstruction of the coronary ostia), although this is rare.

Definitive diagnosis   Transoesophageal echocardiography, thoracic CT scanning and MRI have high sensitivity in the detection of dissections. Thoracic aortography is still required occasionally.

Management

Medical treatment with analgesia and reduction of heart rate and blood pressure with beta-blockers is important. Immediate surgery is required in all patients with acute dissection of the ascending aorta (type A). The ascending aorta is replaced with a prosthetic graft and the false channel is obliterated. Operative mortality, however, remains around 50%. Surgery for distal (type B) dissection is usually reserved for patients developing complications or those with Marfan's syndrome.

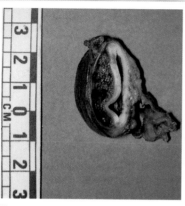

Fig. 192 Dissecting aneurysm (postmortem) with tracking of blood in the media and partial obliteration of the lumen.

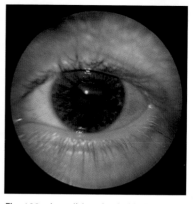

Fig. 193 Lens dislocation in Marfan's syndrome.

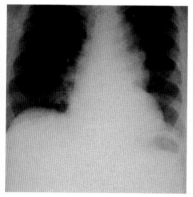

Fig. 194 Chest X-ray showing widened mediastinum.

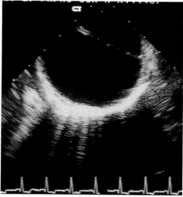

Fig. 195 Transoesophageal echo showing true and false lumens.

Complication of venous thrombosis usually arising in the deep veins of the legs. Some patients postoperatively are at particular risk (e.g. increased age, immobility, malignancy).

Clinical features

Clinical diagnosis lacks both sensitivity and specificity. Symptoms may include dyspnoea on exertion and at rest, pleuritic or central chest pain, haemoptysis and syncope. On examination the patient may be tachypnoeic, using accessory muscles, or have a friction rub, a left parasternal heave, raised venous pressure and tachycardia, or no signs whatsoever.

Investigations

Chest X-ray   Often normal, and findings when present are non-specific, e.g. basal atelectasis. Most helpful in demonstrating another cause for the patient's clinical presentation – pneumothorax, pneumonia, pulmonary oedema, etc.

Electrocardiography   is often normal (>30%) or reveals a sinus tachycardia only. Changes such as $S_1Q_3T_3$ and RBBB are non-specific. The ECG may serve to exclude other possible causes of symptoms, e.g. myocardial infarction.

Lung scanning   Perfusion or ventilation/perfusion scanning is often useful as an initial diagnostic test. Mismatching of ventilation and perfusion with pulmonary embolism is a useful pointer to the diagnosis but can be non-specific.

High resolution CT/CT pulmonary angiography   is now the investigation of choice.

Pulmonary angiography   Reference standard for the diagnosis of pulmonary embolism. Emboli are demonstrated as constant filling defects with a sharp cut off.

Management

Most patients require anticoagulation initially with heparin and subsequently with warfarin. Patients with massive pulmonary embolism may be candidates for more aggressive therapy with thrombolytic agents or pulmonary embolectomy. Fragmentation of an embolus with the tip of a pulmonary catheter can speed dissolution. Prevention of the passage of further clot from the deep venous system may be aided by the insertion of a caval filter.

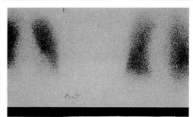

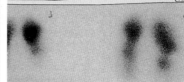

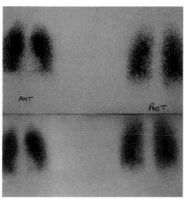

Fig. 196 Normal ventilation (upper) and perfusion (lower) scans.

Fig. 197 Mismatch of ventilation and perfusion with multiple pulmonary emboli.

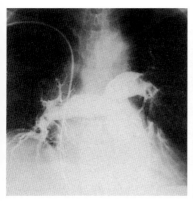

Fig. 198 Pulmonary angiogram showing filling defect and sharp cut-off typical of pulmonary embolism.

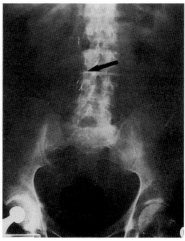

Fig. 199 Intracaval filter in situ.

37 Primary pulmonary hypertension

Pulmonary hypertension is defined by the presence of a high pulmonary artery pressure reflecting increased pulmonary vascular resistance. In many patients no specific cause is identified and the condition is termed primary pulmonary hypertension. The pathology consists of muscular hypertrophy, constriction and hypoplasia of peripheral pulmonary arteries, leading to the development of plexiform lesions.

Clinical features

The condition affects females more than males (ratio 5:1). Patients are usually young (age 15–40) and present with fatigue and exertional syncope, but chest pain or dyspnoea may be predominant. Patients may have evidence of a connective tissue disease with Raynaud's phenomenon and have a malar flush. On examination, patients usually have peripheral but not central cyanosis when at rest. They may have an α wave visible in the venous pulse, a right ventricular heave and, on auscultation, a loud pulmonary component of the second heart sound.

Investigations

Chest X-ray may show cardiomegaly with enlargement of the right-sided chambers, pulmonary artery enlargement with peripheral oligaemia (pruning), and a small aortic knuckle.

Echocardiography demonstrates a dilated right ventricle and paradoxical septal motion. Pulmonary artery pressure can be estimated.

Right heart catheter Confirms diagnosis of pulmonary hypertension with a raised pulmonary artery pressure. Mixed venous oxygen saturation and cardiac output correlate with prognosis

Pulmonary angiography Usually required to exclude large-vessel thromboembolism that might be helped by thromboendarterectomy.

Lung biopsy Definitive diagnostic test, although similar changes can occur in Eisenmenger's complex.

Management

Although spontaneous remission has been reported, the usual tendency is a progressive downhill course with a 10-year survival of less than 25%. Most patients should receive anticoagulants and a trial of vasodilator therapy may be attempted with caution. Thromboendarterectomy or heart–lung transplantation should be considered in selected patients.

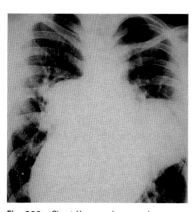

Fig. 200 Chest X-ray: primary pulmonary hypertension with massive proximal pulmonary arteries.

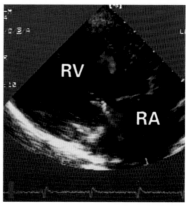

Fig. 201 Right ventricular enlargement on two-dimensional echocardiogram.

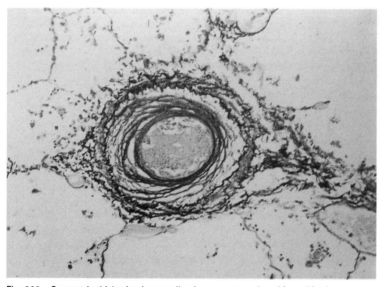

Fig. 202 Concentric thickening in a small pulmonary artery: lung biopsy histology.

75% of cardiac tumours are benign; the most common by far are myxomas but lipomas, fibroelastomas and rhabdomyomas can also occur.

Atrial myxoma

Myxomas are thought to arise from primitive mesenchymal cells. 90% arise in the atria, four times more commonly on the left than the right. They are pedunculated and attached to the interatrial septum at the fossa ovalis. Patients may present at any age. In some the condition is familial. Patients may be asymptomatic or present with symptoms of mitral stenosis, with systemic embolism or constitutional symptoms such as lethargy, fevers, etc. Findings on examination can be similar to those in mitral stenosis. Routine laboratory tests may be abnormal, with normochromic normocytic anaemia, leukocytosis, raised ESR and gammaglobulins. Chest X-ray appearances may resemble those of mitral stenosis, although the left atrial appendage is not so prominent. The tumour may be calcified. Echocardiography is the investigation of choice. Angiography is no longer required but may produce dramatic images. Complete surgical resection is the treatment of choice.

Malignant cardiac tumours

The most common are directly invasive from lung primaries or secondary deposits from elsewhere. Sarcomas are the most common primary cardiac tumours and present with heart failure, arrhythmias and effusions. The prognosis in these patients is extremely poor.

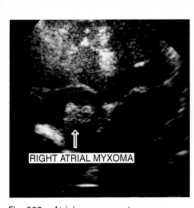

Fig. 203 Atrial myxoma on two-dimensional echo.

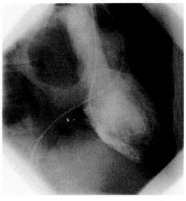

Fig. 204 Atrial myxoma on angiography shown as large filling defect after mitral reflux from LV angiogram.

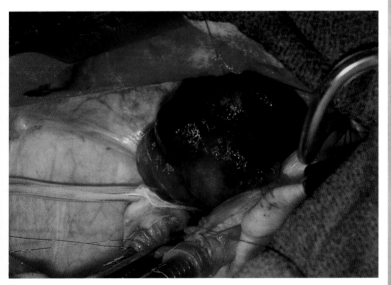

Fig. 205 Removal of atrial myxoma.

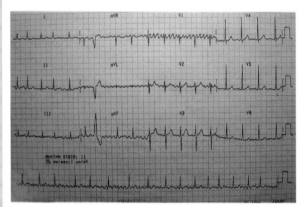

1. A 67-year-old man with a productive cough was brought to Accident and Emergency.

a. What rhythm does this 12-lead ECG show?
b. What is the immediate course of action if haemodynamically compromised?
c. What underlying causes need to be excluded?
d. How should the patient be managed long-term?

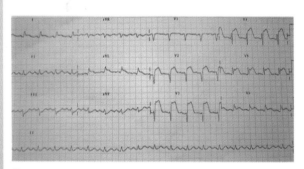

2. This ECG is from a 50-year-old male smoker with chest tightness.

a. What is the diagnosis?
b. What is the immediate treatment?
c. What are the contraindications to this treatment?
d. What risks need to be discussed with the patient?

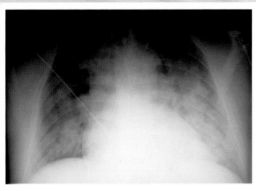

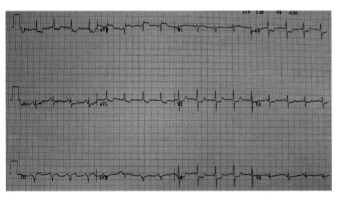

3. A 70-year-old man with severe chest pain of 3 hours duration suddenly became profoundly breathless. A loud pansystolic murmur was easily audible across the praecordium, which had not been previously documented.

a. What does the chest X-ray reveal?
b. What is the differential diagnosis?
c. How can the diagnosis be confirmed?
d. How should this patient be managed?

4. This exercise ECG was taken from a 56-year-old man during stage 2 of the Bruce protocol. He complained of breathlessness and mild tightness across the chest.

a. What does the ECG show?
b. What is the significance of this finding?
c. What are the causes of false positive tests?
d. What are the contraindications to this investigation?

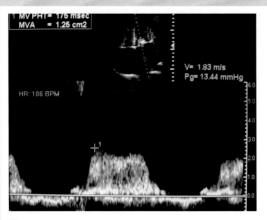

5. This 26-year-old woman, who was 33 weeks pregnant with her first child, complained of breathlessness and haemoptysis.

a. What does the echocardiogram reveal?
b. What other physical findings would be expected?
c. What are the immediate dangers?
d. How should the patient be managed?

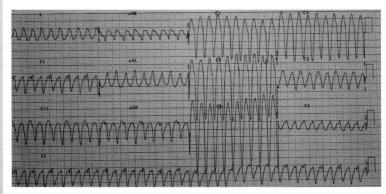

6. This ECG was recorded from a 45-year-old man who suddenly became unwell 4 days after an otherwise uncomplicated myocardial infarction.

a. What does the ECG reveal?
b. What is the immediate management?
c. What medication has prognostic benefit in this situation?
d. What is the definitive management?

7. A 32-year-old drug abuser was admitted with pyrexia and left-sided weakness. A harsh systolic murmur was audible in the aortic area.

a. What does the transoesophageal echocardiogram reveal?
b. What is the likely cause of the weakness?
c. What is the most likely causative agent?
d. What is the treatment strategy?

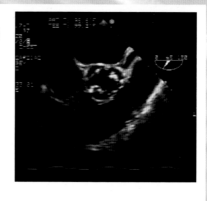

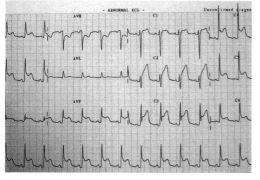

8. A 71-year-old man presented with chest pains and breathlessness. Despite treatment, he became increasingly hypotensive and oliguric. Echocardiography revealed anterolateral akinesia, with estimated ejection fraction of 10%.

a. What does the ECG reveal?
b. Where is the lesion likely to be?
c. What are the treatment options?
d. What is the prognosis?

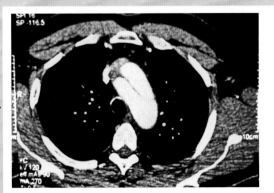

9. A 51-year-old woman was admitted by the general surgeons with epigastric discomfort, radiating into the back. Her blood pressure was 170/100 despite long-term antihypertensive therapy.

a. What abnormality is seen on the CT scan?
b. What is the likely aetiology?
c. How is this condition treated?
d. What are the risks?

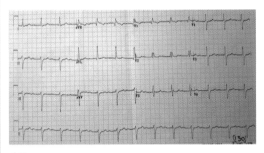

10. An 82-year-old woman was brought to Accident & Emergency with a fractured hip following a fall. She had a history of recurrent fainting spells for some time. She denied chest pains or palpitations. She was taking no regular medication.

a. What abnormalities are seen on the ECG?
b. What is the likely cause of the falls?
c. What is the treatment?
d. What precautions need to be taken preoperatively?

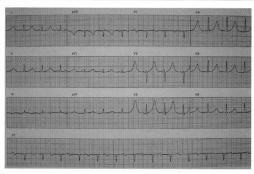

11. A 15-year-old girl was referred to the neurology department following a series of fits. All investigations were normal.

a. What abnormality is shown?
b. What is the likely cause of the fits?
c. What are the causes of this condition?
d. What is the treatment?

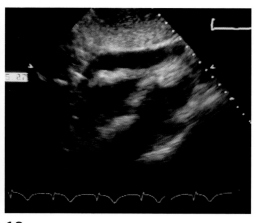

12. A 58-year-old man returned to the UK from a prolonged stay in Pakistan. He complained of a cough and gradually worsening breathlessness.

a. What abnormality is seen on the echo?
b. What is the likely aetiology?
c. How is this treated?
d. What is the cause of the productive cough?

13. A 60-year-old woman with severe peripheral vascular disease was referred for investigation of exertional chest pains.

a. What investigation has been performed and why?
b. What abnormality is shown?
c. What are the causes of false-positive results?
d. What is the next most likely course of action?

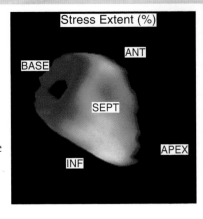

Stress Extent (%)

ANT
BASE
SEPT
APEX
INF

14. A 45-year-old cardiac technician complained of occasional sharp chest pains and irregular palpitations, but was otherwise well. A 12-lead ECG performed by a colleague revealed infrequent unifocal ventricular ectopy.

a. What does the echocardiogram reveal?
b. What physical findings would be expected?
c. Is the diagnosis cause for concern?
d. What therapy is recommended?

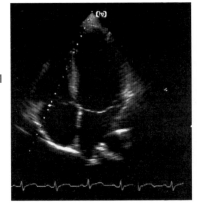

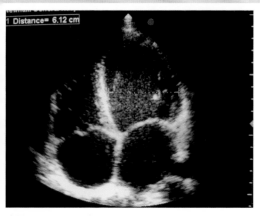

15. A 22-year-old pregnant woman complained of increasing breathlessness and ankle swelling as she entered her 37th week with her first child. Examination revealed an elevated jugular venous pressure and bibasal crepitations.

a. What is the differential diagnosis?
b. What abnormality is seen on the echocardiogram?
c. What is the treatment?
d. What is the prognosis?

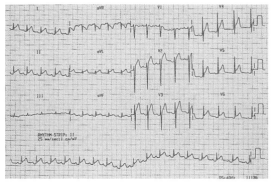

16. This 55-year-old man returned to casualty 4 weeks after an uncomplicated myocardial infarction. The pain was unlike that with the infarct, and changed with posture. All his blood tests were normal except for an elevated ESR at 97 mm/h.

a. What presumed pathophysiology causes this ECG appearance?
b. How often is this complication seen?
c. What is the underlying pathology?
d. How is it treated?

17. A 35-year-old man was referred to the rheumatology outpatient clinic with mild pyrexia and generalized aches and pains. The day before he had experienced sudden loss of vision in the left eye, which spontaneously resolved within the hour. Examination was normal, except for a soft, low-pitched diastolic murmur.

a. What abnormality is seen on the echocardiogram?
b. What is the cause of the constitutional symptoms?
c. What is the cause of the transient blindness?
d. What is the treatment and prognosis?

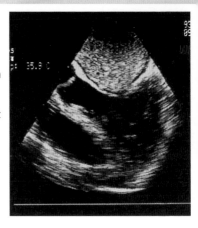

18. A 29-year-old fitness instructor collapsed during an aerobics class. He rapidly regained consciousness and was reluctant to attend hospital. He had experienced several similar episodes, associated with exercise, as had his brother.

a. What is the abnormal feature of this echocardiogram?
b. What is the likely underlying cause of collapse?
c. How is the condition inherited?
d. What are the occupational implications of this diagnosis?

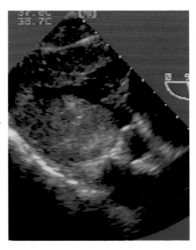

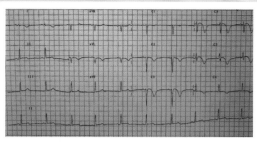

19. A 52-year-old woman presented with exercise-induced chest pain. Examination was normal except for mild epigastric tenderness. Her only significant past medical was chronic pancreatitis. She was a non-smoker and did not drink alcohol. ECG revealed ischaemic features and serum troponin I was positive at 1.8. Her plasma sodium was low at 125.

a. What is the probable cause of her chest pain?
b. What risk factor could explain the low sodium?
c. What is the immediate treatment?
d. Do her family require further screening?

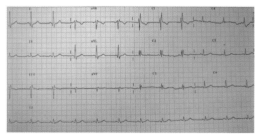

20. A 35-year-old man was referred with increasing breathlessness and intermittent palpitations. Clinical examination revealed a split second heart sound.

a. What abnormality is seen on the ECG?
b. What is the probable diagnosis?
c. How is this confirmed?
d. What are the treatment options?

21. A 22-year-old basketball player suddenly developed chest pain during a match. He rapidly deteriorated and was markedly hypotensive on arrival in Accident & Emergency.

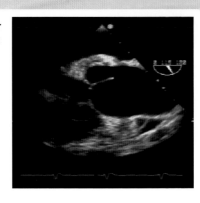

a. What investigation has been performed and what abnormality is revealed?
b. What is the probable underlying condition in this case?
c. What is the immediate treatment?
d. What is the prognosis?

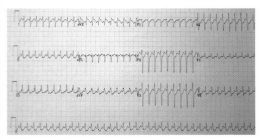

22. A 27-year-old teacher presented to Accident & Emergency with sudden onset palpitations and breathlessness. She had experienced similar symptoms on numerous occasions, which had usually terminated with coughing.

a. What does the ECG reveal?
b. Why did coughing usually help?
c. What is the immediate therapy?
d. What are the long-term options?

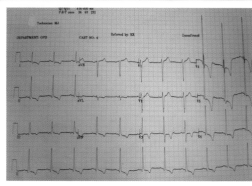

23. A 60-year-old man with no cardiac risk factors was referred for investigation of breathlessness and two episodes of exercise-induced syncope. An ejection systolic murmur was heard throughout the praecordium.

a. What is the ECG finding?
b. What are the common causes of this appearance?
c. What is the likely diagnosis in this case?
d. What investigations will be required?

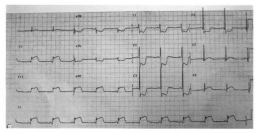

24. A 19-year-old man was found collapsed in a night club. On arrival in Accident & Emergency he complained of severe chest pains. He received thrombolytic therapy shortly afterwards, with eventual resolution of pain and ECG changes. The rise in creatinine kinase was minimal and subsequent coronary catheterization was normal.

a. What is the ECG abnormality?
b. What other risk factor must be considered in this case?
c. How do you explain the appearance of the coronary arteries?
d. What is the prognosis?

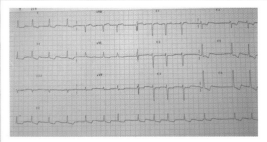

25. A 78-year-old woman was admitted to a surgical ward with a long history of nausea and vomiting. She had a history of atrial fibrillation that was controlled on medication. A cardiology opinion was sought prior to elective laparotomy.

a. What abnormality is seen on the ECG?
b. What are the causes of this appearance?
c. What is the probable diagnosis and how can it be confirmed?
d. What is the treatment?

26. A 30-year-old man was found collapsed outside his home in the early hours and was taken to Accident & Emergency. He had taken an unknown quantity of atenolol, paracetamol and alcohol.

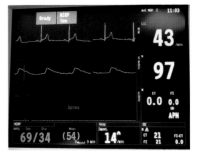

a. What potentially worrying features are seen on the resuscitation monitor?
b. Which two simple bedside tests are urgently required?
c. What immediate action is required?
d. What medication would you prescribe?

27. A 35-year-old man had been troubled by recurrent supraventricular arrhythmia for many years. He was asthmatic, and intolerant of flecainide.

a. What procedure is being performed?
b. What are the common indications?
c. What complications can occur?
d. What is the cure rate for this condition?

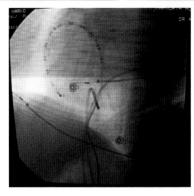

28. A 28-year-old woman complained of aching joints and fever, which had been gradually worsening for the past few months. Clinical examination revealed polyarthritis, a generalized rash and splenomegaly. No murmur was detected.

a. What does the echocardiogram reveal?
b. What is the diagnosis?
c. What other cardiac complications are seen with this condition?
d. How is it treated?

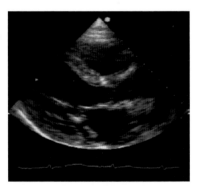

29. A 78-year-old man was admitted following a collapse at home. He had suffered a myocardial infarction the previous year, which was complicated by complete heart block, ventricular fibrillation and left ventricular failure. An implantable cardioverter defibrillator was inserted at the time. Shortly after admission he suffered a further collapse and a defibrillator shock was delivered.

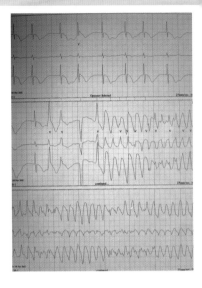

a. What abnormalities are seen on the telemetry print-out?
b. What is the probable cause of the collapse?
c. How should this patient be managed?
d. What is the prognosis?

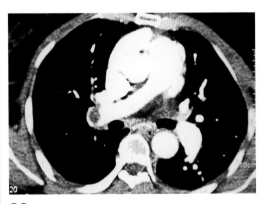

30. A 70-year-old woman presented to Accident & Emergency complaining of sudden-onset chest pain and breathlessness. Her oxygen saturation was 85% despite supplementary oxygen.

a. What abnormalities are seen on the CT scan?
b. What would you expect to see on the chest X-ray?
c. What is the probable diagnosis?
d. What is the treatment?

31. A 65-year-old man collapsed on the coronary care unit 3 days after an otherwise uncomplicated myocardial infarction. Cardiac arrest was confirmed and cardiopulmonary resuscitation commenced.

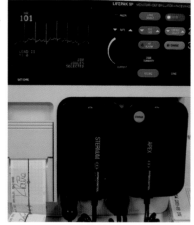

a. What does the ECG monitor reveal?
b. What is the term used for this type of cardiac arrest?
c. What are the eight recognized causes?
d. Which of these causes may be relevant in this case?

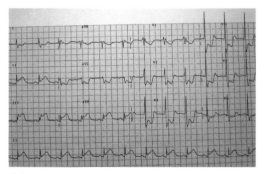

32. A 65-year old man was treated for a myocardial infarction. 24 hours later, he became increasingly hypotensive and oliguric. His chest was clear to auscultation. A central venous catheter was inserted, and CVP was measured at 25cm H2O.

a. What does the ECG reveal?
b. Which artery is likely to be responsible?
c. How do you explain the absence of pulmonary oedema despite an elevated CVP?
d. What is the immediate treatment?

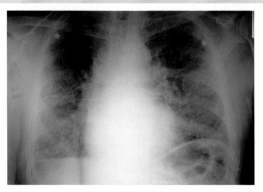

33. A 57-year-old woman was referred by the endocrinology team with increasing breathlessness. She had recently commenced thyroxine therapy and was taking medication for long-standing palpitations, although she could not recall the name of the tablet.

a. What abnormality is seen on the chest X-ray?
b. What is the probable identity of the unknown medication?
c. What are the other side effects?
d. What action should be taken?

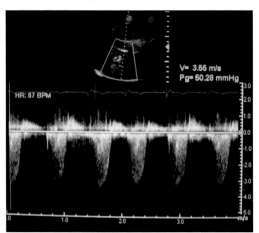

34. A 34-year-old woman with systemic sclerosis was referred to the cardiology department with increasing breathlessness. Examination revealed a loud second heart sound and a quiet pansystolic murmur heard at the left sternal edge.

a. What abnormalities can be seen on the echocardiogram?
b. What is the diagnosis?
c. What other clinical features are seen in this condition?
d. How is this condition managed?

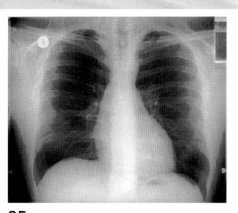

35. A 29-year-old man was referred to the cardiology department with difficult-to-control hypertension despite four antihypertensive agents. Examination was unremarkable, apart from a soft systolic murmur in the aortic area and a rumbling murmur heard over the chest posteriorly.

a. What abnormality is seen on the chest X-ray?
b. What is the likely diagnosis?
c. What other clinical features would be expected?
d. How is the diagnosis confirmed?

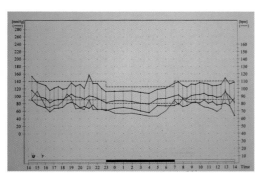

36. A 28-year-old woman was found to be hypertensive during a gym medical. She was previously well, with no significant past medical history. The blood pressure measured in clinic was 165/95 mmHg. A 24-hour blood pressure recording was undertaken prior to consideration of treatment.

a. What does the above 24-hour recording reveal?
b. Is this condition benign?
c. What further investigations are required?
d. What is the first-line strategy?

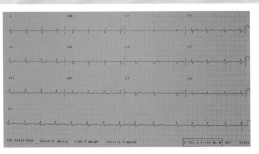

37. A 75-year-old man was admitted with increasing breathlessness. His venous pressure was elevated, and a gallop rhythm was audible over the praecordium. Leg swelling and ascites were also present. Peripheral neuropathy was also detected.

a. What is the ECG abnormality?
b. What is the probable diagnosis?
c. What other non-cardiac features are seen in this condition?
d. How is the diagnosis confirmed?

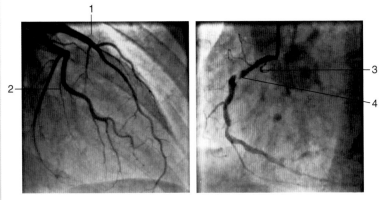

38. A 53-year-old man underwent coronary angiography following a history of exercise-induced chest pains and a positive exercise tolerance test.

a. What structure is labelled 1?
b. What structure is labelled 2?
c. What structure is labelled 3?
d. What abnormality is labelled 4?

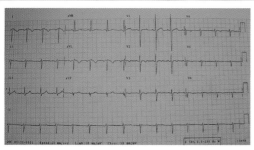

39. A 26-year-old man was referred to the cardiology clinic because of an incidental ECG abnormality. He suffered very frequent and often severe chest infections, for which he received antibiotics, but was otherwise well. His apex was impalpable and heart sounds were very quiet.

a. What does the ECG show?
b. Explain the physical findings?
c. What is the diagnosis?
d. What is the cause of the chest infection?

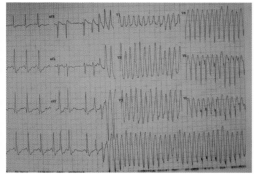

40. A 76-year-old man was recovering from a myocardial infarction on the coronary care unit. His past medical history included mild hypertension. Whilst cleaning his teeth, the following is seen.

a. What abnormality is seen on the ECG telemetry?
b. In this scenario, what are the two most common causes?
c. What is the management?

Answers

1.
- a. Atrial fibrillation with a ventricular rate of approximately 120 beats per minute.
- b. Urgent sedation and synchronized DC cardioversion.
- c. Sepsis, hyperthyroidism, valvular heart disease, ischaemic heart disease, cardiomyopathy and alcohol abuse.
- d. Anticoagulation with warfarin to achieve an INR of 2–3 to prevent cerebral thromboembolism. Spontaneous return to sinus rhythm may occur with correction of the underlying cause in some cases, such as sepsis. Attempts can be made to restore sinus rhythm via either elective DC cardioversion or the use of drugs (amiodarone or flecainide). If AF is accepted, drugs such as digoxin, beta-blockers or calcium antagonists can be used to control the ventricular rate.

2.
- a. Anterior myocardial infarction.
- b. Oxygen, analgesia, aspirin, urgent intravenous thrombolysis, heparin and beta blockade.
- c. Bleeding disorders, recent haemorrhage (gastrointestinal, intracerebral, heavy menstrual), recent surgery, aortic dissection, severe hypertension, severe liver disease.
- d. Intracerebral haemorrhage that can be fatal (approximately 1%). Major bleeding that may require transfusion or surgery. Nausea, vomiting and allergic reactions.

3.
- a. Widespread alveolar shadowing with upper lobe blood diversion, consistent with acute pulmonary oedema.
- b. Acute myocardial infarction that has been complicated by either mitral valve rupture or ventricular septal defect.
- c. Urgent echocardiography with colour flow Doppler.
- d. Insertion of intra-aortic balloon pump may provide temporary stabilization while definitive corrective surgery is arranged. There is no role for medical management.

4.
- a. Down-sloping ST segment depression of approximately 3 mm in the anterolateral leads.
- b. Given that this appearance is associated with pain, the probability of coronary artery disease is high.
- c. Hyperventilation, anaemia, mitral valve prolapse, left ventricular hypertrophy, hypertrophic cardiomyopathy and certain drugs, particularly antidepressants.
- d. Aortic stenosis, severe left ventricular failure, severe angina (especially with previous rest pain), myo/pericarditis and complete heart block.

148

5. *a.* The continuous wave Doppler reveals a flow pattern indicative of mitral stenosis.

 b. Atrial fibrillation, tapping apex beat, opening snap with a low-pitched rumbling diastolic murmur heard in the left lateral position with held expiration.

 c. This valve lesion leads to a fixed cardiac output state, which prevents the patient from accommodating to the wide fluctuations in plasma volume that can occur during delivery, predisposing to both hypotension and pulmonary oedema.

 d. This particular patient underwent emergency mitral balloon valvuloplasty followed by elective caesarean section. Formal valve replacement surgery was undertaken at a later stage.

6. *a.* Broad complex, regular tachycardia with a rate above 200 beats per minute. There is concordance and extreme axis deviation. In the context of a recent myocardial infarction, the most likely diagnosis is ventricular tachycardia.

 b. If haemodynamically compromised, urgent sedation and synchronized DC cardioversion is the treatment of choice. Otherwise, amiodarone or lidocaine (lignocaine) may be successful in terminating the arrhythmia.

 c. Aspirin, beta-blockers, ACE inhibitors, statins and aldosterone antagonists are the only prognostically beneficial medication in this situation. No clear survival advantage has been observed with any antiarrhythmic agent other than beta-blockers.

 d. Coronary heart disease is the probable substrate for the arrhythmia, so invasive imaging of the coronary tree and revascularization as required is recommended. Secondary arrhythmia prophylaxis is essential and only effectively provided by the use of an implantable cardioverter defibrillator (ICD).

7. *a.* A mass is seen in the region of the aortic valve.

 b. Mycotic embolus is most probable.

 c. Right-sided staphylococcal infections are commonly seen in intravenous drug addicts.

 d. Prolonged high-dose intravenous antibiotics to sterilize the valve. If substantial damage has been sustained, replacement surgery can then be performed. Emergency surgery is required with sudden valvular failure or failure of medical therapy. The risk of replacement valve infection is greater when surgery is undertaken without prior eradication of infection.

8. *a.* Anterolateral ST segment elevation consistent with extensive myocardial infarction.

 b. Left main stem or proximal left anterior descending artery.

 c. Treatment includes aggressive attempts at urgent revascularization including thrombolysis, PCI or surgery. Inotropic support or intra-aortic balloon pump insertion may provide temporary stabilization. Dual chamber pacing is also of benefit in the presence of complete heart block.

    d. Despite recent advances, the 30-day mortality for cardiogenic shock following a myocardial infarction is 90%.

9.
    a. A dissection flap is seen within the aortic arch, with contrast in both the true and false lumen.
    b. Hypertension is the likely aetiology.
    c. Aggressive control of blood pressure is required followed by an assessment of the suitability for surgical repair.
    d. Stroke, myocardial infarction, paraplegia and death are the most serious complications.

10.
    a. First-degree AV block, left axis deviation, right bundle branch block (trifascicular block).
    b. Intermittent complete heart block and symptomatic bradycardia.
    c. Insertion of a permanent pacemaker.
    d. Insertion of a temporary pacing wire.

11.
    a. The QT interval is prolonged, at over 500 ms. The normal upper limit is 460 ms for women, 440 ms for men.
    b. Long QT predisposes to polymorphic ventricular tachycardia (*torsade de pointes*), which may be associated with loss of cardiac output and can degenerate into ventricular fibrillation.
    c. It may be due to an inherited abnormality of the cardiac ion channel function (ion channelopathy). In such cases a family history of similar episodes or sudden death may be present. Alternatively, certain drugs (amiodarone, cisapride, terfenadine) may be responsible. Hypokalaemia, hypocalcaemia and hypomagnesaemia are also known precipitants.
    d. In acquired cases, identification and withdrawal of the offending agent is required. Beta-blockers and possibly also implantable cardioverter defibrillator insertion would be recommended in inherited cases.

12.
    a. A large pericardial effusion is seen.
    b. Tuberculosis is most likely given this patient's travel history and respiratory symptoms. Such a large effusion must have accumulated slowly, in keeping with a chronic condition. Malignancy is another possible aetiology.
    c. Treatment of the underlying cause is indicated in most chronic pericardial effusions. Drainage of the collection is performed only for diagnostic purposes or in the presence of haemodynamic compromise.
    d. A cough can occur as a result of the distended pericardium exerting pressure on the overlying phrenic nerve. Respiratory involvement of the underlying aetiology may also be responsible.

13.
    a. A stress thallium scan, presumably in place of an exercise tolerance test due to claudication.
    b. Anteroapical ischaemia.

c. Left bundle branch block, valve disease, cardiomyopathy, previous cardiac surgery and breast implants.

d. Coronary angiography, with a view to revascularization. Gaining vascular access may be difficult, given the peripheral vascular disease.

14.
a. Prolapse of the anterior mitral valve leaflet.

b. An irregular pulse due to the ectopy; a pansystolic murmur, depending on the severity of the mitral regurgitation; and a possible midsystolic click caused by the tensing chordae of the prolapsing leaflet.

c. This condition is seen in up to 10% of the normal population. Rare case reports of sudden death and stroke do exist, but the condition is essentially benign.

d. Antibiotic prophylaxis for dental treatment if the prolapse is associated with a murmur.

15.
a. Minor ankle swelling and breathlessness may be physiological in pregnancy but the elevated JVP and pulmonary oedema are abnormal. Peripartum cardiomyopathy, pericardial effusion/tamponade and pulmonary embolism should all be considered.

b. A globally dilated heart consistent with peripartum cardiomyopathy.

c. Rapid elective delivery and ACE inhibitors are often the only treatment necessary, and recovery can be complete. In severe cases, ventricular assist devices and transplantation may be required.

d. Generally good in mild-moderate cases.

16.
a. Dressler's syndrome or postinfarction pericarditis (and occasionally pleuritis). Chest discomfort is typically pericarditic/pleuritic. Small pericardial or pleural effusions are seen, although tamponade is uncommon. A similar picture follows cardiac surgery.

b. It affects approximately 5% of all myocardial infarctions.

c. Infarcted myocardium becomes antigenic, leading to subsequent autoimmune inflammation.

d. Essentially self-limiting although symptomatic benefit may be provided with non-steroidal anti-inflammatory drugs.

17.
a. A rounded mass is seen that fills the right atrium. It most likely represents an atrial myxoma.

b. Non-specific symptoms are often due to tumour production of inflammatory mediators.

c. Retinal artery embolism is the most likely cause, usually dislodged thrombus that collects on the tumour surface.

d. Treatment is surgical excision, which is curative in most instances. Incomplete resection may lead to recurrence.

18.
a. The septum and posterior wall are grossly thickened. The appearance is that of hypertrophic cardiomyopathy.

b. Ventricular tachycardia is the most likely arrhythmia, leading to transient loss of cardiac output.

c. The inheritance is autosomal dominant in most cases, with sporadic gene mutations in the remainder.

d. Extreme physical activity should be avoided in all cases of exercise induced syncope.

19. a. An acute coronary syndrome is most probable given the ECG changes and positive troponin.

b. Severe hyperlipidaemia is a well recognized cause of pseudohyponatraemia.

c. Aspirin, clopidogrel, low-molecular-weight heparin in the first instance. A beta-blocker, ACE inhibitor and statin would all be beneficial over the course of the inpatient stay. Cardiac catheterization would be indicated in this case.

d. In all suspected cases of familial hypercholesterolaemia, screening of first -degree relatives is advisable, with referral to a lipidologist as required.

20. a. Right bundle branch block.

b. Atrial septal defect.

c. Transoesophageal echocardiography is required to visualize the defect and assess the degree of right ventricular volume overloading and pulmonary pressures. Right heart catheterization is usually performed, and coronary angiography in those over the age of 40.

d. Increasing symptoms, cerebroembolic events and left-to-right shunting of >2:1 are all indications for closure. This can either performed surgically (with coronary revascularization if required) or percutaneously in selected cases.

21. a. Trans-oesophageal echocardiography (TOE) reveals a dissection flap within the aorta.

b. The most likely underlying condition is Marfan's syndrome. This collagen vascular disease is inherited in an autosomal dominant manner. Other features include a thin, tall habitus with arm-span greater than height, arachnodactyly, high arched palate and lens dislocation. Cystic medial necrosis leads to vascular weakness, and dissection of the aortic arch is a common complication.

c. Immediate fluid resuscitation and urgent surgical repair.

d. Unfortunately, the prognosis is poor once dissection has occurred. Prophylactic aortic root replacement is therefore performed in most patients once the diameter has exceeded 5.5 cm.

22. a. Narrow complex tachycardia with a rate of approximately 250 beats/min, consistent with an atrioventricular node re-entrant tachycardia (AVNRT).

b. Coughing mimics the Valsalva manoeuvre, raising vagal tone and consequently slowing AV conduction. This may well terminate the arrhythmia. Sneezing, blowing, retching, iced water and gently massaging the carotid artery can also increase vagal tone.

    c. Intravenous adenosine creates temporary AV block (<10 s) and is commonly used in this condition. Caution needs to be taken with asthmatics, as bronchospasm may occur. An intravenous calcium channel blocker (e.g. verapamil) can be used, with caution.

    d. Beta-blockers and class Ic agents such as flecainide are effective in suppressing such arrhythmia but are associated with side effects. In all cases, radiofrequency ablation offers a permanent solution at low risk.

23. a. Left ventricular hypertrophy with lateral strain pattern. The sum of the S wave in V1 and the R wave in V_6 is >35 mm (Sokolow criterion).

    b. Hypertension, left ventricular outflow obstruction (aortic stenosis), athletic training.

    c. Given the absence of hypertension and the detection of a systolic murmur, aortic stenosis is the likely diagnosis.

    d. The diagnosis can be confirmed by echocardiography. Because valve replacement may be required, cardiac catheterization is indicated, as simultaneous coronary revascularisation can be performed. Renal function, carotid Doppler studies and a dental assessment are all required.

24. a. ST elevation affecting the inferior leads (II, III, aVF), in keeping with an acute inferior myocardial infarction.

    b. Use of illicit drugs, particularly cocaine, must be considered in young patients without apparent risk factors for coronary disease.

    c. Cocaine can induce intense coronary vasospasm, which may lead to myocardial infarction even in the absence of coronary disease. It is also arrhythmogenic and can induce life-threatening ventricular arrhythmia.

    d. Generally good, provided further drug use is avoided.

25. a. Lateral ST segment depression with a 'reversed tick' appearance.

    b. This is the classical appearance of digoxin toxicity, although a similar pattern is seen with lateral ischaemia, and strain pattern associated with left ventricular hypertrophy.

    c. This patient complains of nausea and vomiting, and is receiving treatment for atrial fibrillation. The symptoms are consistent with digoxin toxicity, possibly compounded by hypokalaemia from the vomiting. An urgent plasma digoxin level is required (normal range 1–2 mmol/l).

    d. Supportive measures, including fluid and electrolyte replacement as well as withdrawal of the offending digoxin, should suffice in most situations, although specific antidigoxin medication is available.

26. a. He has a sinus bradycardia and is hypotensive.

    b. Core body temperature and blood glucose.

    c. Oxygen and intravenous access. Hypoglycaemia should be corrected and warm fluid resuscitation should be commenced if hypothermic.

    d. Glucagon is recommended for the treatment of beta-blocker overdose. Atropine and isoprenaline are often ineffective. Temporary cardiac pacing may be required. N-acetyl cysteine is given to minimize hepatic damage.

27. *a.* This is a picture taken during an electrophysiological study. Various recording catheters have been placed within the heart. Once the source of the arrhythmia has been identified, it can be destroyed using radio-frequency energy delivered by the ablation catheter.
b. Any patient with recurrent arrhythmia should be referred for consideration of ablation.
c. Complications include bleeding/haematoma at the puncture site, AV node damage, cardiac perforation, embolic stroke and death. All these are now very rare.
d. Cure is now available for most supraventricular arrhythmias.

28. *a.* A small rounded mass is seen on the mitral valve leaflet.
b. This patient has systemic lupus erythematosus. The valve lesion is termed Libman–Sachs endocarditis and is seen in up to 50% of cases. Although the vegetation may be large, valve destruction is uncommon, unlike infective endocarditis.
c. Sinus tachycardia, pericarditis (with effusion/tamponade), myocarditis and coronary vasculitis have all been reported.
d. Cardiac manifestations often improve with treatment of the underlying condition with steroids and disease-modifying agents. In severe cases, valve replacement surgery may be required.

29. *a.* Several paced beats are seen, followed by a ventricular ectopic beat that initiates ventricular tachycardia.
b. Loss of cardiac output secondary to ventricular tachycardia or ventricular fibrillation.
c. He requires admission to the coronary care unit with ICD interrogation. If multiple appropriate shocks are being received, adequate sedation and analgesia is needed. Underlying causes such as electrolyte imbalance and ischaemia should be identified and treated. Intravenous antiarrhythmic drugs such as sotalol, lidocaine (lignocaine) or amiodarone may be required.
d. Severe heart failure (NYHA class III/IV) carries a poor prognosis, with annual mortality rates of 30–40%. Death is usually due to ventricular arrhythmia.

30. *a.* A round mass is seen within the pulmonary artery.
b. Essentially normal. Reduced vascular markings may be seen over the painful region.
c. A large pulmonary embolism.
d. Analgesia and oxygen are required immediately. Anticoagulation is required, with heparin initially, then eventually warfarin. In severe cases, intravenous thrombolysis may be required.

31. *a.* Sinus rhythm with a rate of 100 beats/min.
b. Pulseless electrical activity (PEA).

32.
  a. ST segment elevation in the inferior leads, with a dominant R wave in V1.
  b. Right coronary artery, particularly the posterior descending branch.
  c. The pattern of ECG changes with hypotension and oliguria, and elevated CVP is in keeping with a right ventricular infarction. Pulmonary oedema occurs with impairment of left ventricular function.
  d. Fluid resuscitation is required in the first instance to restore blood pressure and urine output. Thereafter, standard treatment as for myocardial infarction.

33.
  a. Widespread pulmonary fibrosis. The heart size is normal.
  b. The combination of thyroid abnormalities and pulmonary fibrosis suggests that this patient may be taking amiodarone, probably for control of atrial fibrillation.
  c. Corneal deposits (reversible), photosensitivity, hypo- and hyperthyroidism, pneumonitis, neuropathy and hepatotoxicity.
  d. The medication should be withdrawn and replaced with another anti-arrhythmic if required. Many of the side effects, however, are permanent.

34.
  a. Continuous wave Doppler measurement across the tricuspid valve estimates a pulmonary artery pressure of approximately 50 mmHg.
  b. Secondary pulmonary hypertension is a recognized complication of connective tissue disease.
  c. Cyanosis, clubbing (if long-standing), prominent 'a' wave in the jugular venous waveform, right ventricular heave, loud pulmonary second sound, tricuspid and pulmonary regurgitation murmurs.
  d. The condition often mirrors the severity of the underlying condition. In both secondary and primary pulmonary hypertension, anticoagulation and vasodilators form the mainstay of therapy. Ultimately, heart–lung transplantation may be required.

35.
  a. Notching of the posterior edges of the lower ribs.
  b. Coarctation of the aorta should be suspected in this case. The praecordial murmur may be due to a concomitant bicuspid aortic valve or turbulent flow around the region of the coarctation. Collateral blood flow within intercostal arteries leads to the murmur heard posteriorly.
  c. Hypertension, diminished femoral pulse, radio-femoral delay and signs of bicuspid aortic valve.
  d. The lesion can be visualized using MRI or aortography, where the gradient of the lesion can be measured.

36.
  a. The blood pressure appears to be within the normal range during the 24-hour period. As the consistently abnormal readings are only

Before 32:
  c. Hypoxia, hypothermia, hypovolaemia, cardiac tamponade, pulmonary embolism, tension pneumothorax, electrolyte imbalance and drug overdose.
  d. Tamponade following myocardial rupture is the most likely. Treatment would include needle pericardiocentesis and emergency surgery, although the mortality in this situation is considerable.

observed when measured manually, this situation is termed 'white-coat hypertension'.

b. The prevalence of end-organ damage (left ventricular hypertrophy, retinopathy, nephropathy) is less than in the consistently hypertensive population but, even in such borderline cases, the risk of cardiovascular mortality is higher than the normotensive population, so intervention will probably be required.

c. Routine biochemistry, including renal function, thyroid function and 9 am cortisol. Chest X-ray, electrocardiogram, echocardiogram, urinalysis and urine microscopy are required to assess end-organ damage. An abdominal ultrasound is indicated if renal pathology is suspected. If phaeochromocytoma is a possibility, urinary catecholamines should be measured.

d. Non-pharmacological measures such as weight loss, aerobic exercise and reduced-salt diet should be instituted, prior to commencing drug therapy.

37. a. Low voltage complexes are seen throughout.

b. Cardiac amyloidosis and pericardial effusion cause reduced voltage recordings. The clinical scenario of biventricular failure with sensory impairment makes amyloidosis possible.

c. Macroglossia, hepatosplenomegaly, peripheral neuropathy, nephropathy and haematological abnormalities.

d. Serum amyloid protein (SAP) scan or rectal biopsy (with Congo red stain).

38. a. Left anterior descending (LAD) artery.

b. Left circumflex (LCX) artery.

c. Right coronary artery.

d. Severe stenosis of proximal right coronary artery.

39. a. The QRS voltages diminish rather than increase across the chest leads and the polarity is reversed in leads I and aVR.

b. This man has dextrocardia, with the heart situated on the right side of the thorax.

c. Kartagener's syndrome.

d. Bronchiectasis.

40. a. Sudden onset of a broad complex tachycardia.

b. Ventricular tachycardia and muscle artefact (as in this case).

c. Only the former requires treatment, with defibrillation (200 J, 200 J, 360 J).

Index